Disruptive Mood
Irritability in Children
and Adolescents

Disruptive Mood
Irritability in Children and Adolescents

Argyris Stringaris

Institute of Psychiatry Psychology and Neuroscience,
King's College London and Mood Disorder Clinic
for Young people, Maudsley Hospital

and

Eric Taylor

Institute of Psychiatry Psychology and Neuroscience,
King's College London

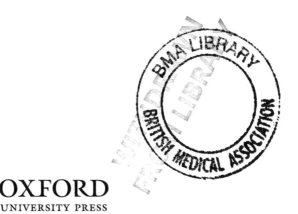
OXFORD
UNIVERSITY PRESS

OXFORD
UNIVERSITY PRESS

Great Clarendon Street, Oxford, OX2 6DP,
United Kingdom

Oxford University Press is a department of the University of Oxford.
It furthers the University's objective of excellence in research, scholarship,
and education by publishing worldwide. Oxford is a registered trade mark of
Oxford University Press in the UK and in certain other countries

Published in the United States of America by Oxford University Press
198 Madison Avenue, New York, NY 10016, United States of America

British Library Cataloguing in Publication Data
Data available

Library of Congress Control Number: 2014953672

ISBN 978-0-19-967454-1

Printed in Great Britain by
Clays Ltd, St Ives plc

Acknowledgements

Professor Taylor gratefully acknowledges the support of the Medical Research Council UK and the Wellcome Trust. Dr Stringaris is grateful for the support from the Wellcome Trust and from the National Institute of Health Research Biomedical Research Centre.

Contents

About the authors

Argyris Stringaris, MD, PhD, MRCPsych, is a clinician scientist studying mood across human development. He trained in psychiatry at the Maudsley Hospital in London, received his PhD at the Institute of Psychiatry at King's College London, and was a Clinical Research Fellow at the National Institute of Mental Health (NIMH) in the USA. He is a Consultant Child and Adolescent Psychiatrist (Attending Physician) with the Mood Disorder Team for Young People at the Maudsley Hospital and a Senior Lecturer at the Institute of Psychiatry, King's College London.

Eric Taylor, MB, FRCP, FRCPsych(Hon), FMedSci has researched, taught, and practised child neuropsychiatry for some 40 years. At The Maudsley Hospital in London he introduced and evaluated a range of treatments, became a director, and is now an honorary consultant. At the Institute of Psychiatry of King's College London he published many research papers and several textbooks and guidelines for practice; he was Head of the Department of Child and Adolescent Psychiatry and is now an Emeritus Professor.

Chapter 1

Irritability: overview and introduction

Children with severe irritability present very often to child mental health services, and there is continuing argument about how to help these young people and their families. To recognize the needs of children with severe irritability, a new condition based on it has been brought into the diagnostic scheme of the fifth edition of the American Psychiatric Association's *Diagnostic and Statistical Manual of Mental Disorders* (DSM-5), the classification system for psychiatric disorders used worldwide. We have written the present book to bring together scientific and clinical knowledge from several sources and help clinicians to understand the origins and management of irritable states in children and adolescents. Our overall perspective is that clinical irritability is best seen as an emotional extreme:

♦ Irritability is a trait of excessive anger—excessive in frequency, duration, intensity, ease of elicitation, and/or uncontrollability. In Chapter 2 we define the terms used more closely. In Chapter 3 we describe the assessment of irritability.

♦ Irritability can lead to aggression towards other people, but very often does not (and there are many other causes of aggression). Researchers and clinicians sometimes regard irritability purely as a matter of disruptive behaviour. This can lead to neglect of the emotional aspects. Chapter 4 describes the early development of the emotion of anger, and the reasons for individual differences in its qualities. Chapter 5 goes on to its prevalence and the course of irritability over time. A central point is that the key risks it imposes for adult life are mood disorders, such as depression, and impaired adaptive function.

♦ Irritability can occur in several different disorders with overlapping diagnostic definitions that often occur together: this can lead to confusion amongst clinicians. Chapters 7–12 deal with the differences in presentation in different psychological disorders, such as attention deficit/hyperactivity disorder (ADHD), autism, and mood disorders, and with the evidence base for treatment.

- Confusion is all the more likely because of current controversies about the boundaries of diagnoses in the different mood disorders. Chapters 10 and 12 address issues about bipolar disorder and the new condition of disruptive mood dysregulation disorder (DMDD), and emphasize the importance of distinguishing between episodic and chronic courses.

- Irritability has neurological as well as psychosocial roots. Chapter 6 indicates some neuropsychological hypotheses about its pathogenesis, but there is too little evidence at the moment for a full theoretical account. Chapter 13 gives an account of brain disease, injury, and disability as influences on irritability. Chapter 14 then draws on previous chapters to summarize recommendations—which necessarily go beyond the evidence base—about how clinicians can navigate the diagnostic complexity and provide useful treatment.

Despite its frequency, irritability has only recently become a focus for research in its own right, and much of the research has not yet been integrated into mainstream clinical thinking. This book discusses some of the core questions:

- *Being irritable is normal: why should irritability be a topic for clinicians in mental health?* Many things that are usually normative, from blood pressure to sadness, can be problematic at the extremes. High blood pressure and persistent sadness are considered pathological, not least because they carry adverse consequences for the individual. Personality and temperament theorists view variations in the levels of irritability as part of inter-individual variation in normative traits, yet it is also recognized that high levels of such traits can put individuals at risk for psychiatric disorders and social maladjustment. This also seems to be the case for irritability. Chapter 5 describes in detail follow-up studies that show irritability to be predictive of adverse outcomes, including psychiatric disorders and social maladjustment, up to 30 years later.

- *Is irritability just a non-specific problem, relating to psychiatry only as fever does to general medicine?* Irritability can indeed occur as part of a number of other psychiatric symptoms and disorders, ranging from depression and generalized anxiety to oppositional–defiant disorder (ODD). Nevertheless, findings from several studies over the past decade suggest that emotional problems, particularly depressive disorders and generalized anxiety, are the long-term outcomes of irritability (Chapter 5). These findings are in keeping with the view that irritability is a mood manifestation and that it shares common risks, and possibly outcomes, with depressive disorders. This view will be discussed further in the chapters on potential mechanisms for irritability (Chapters 6 and 11).

♦ *Should irritability be seen as primarily a disruptive symptom, a characteristic of children with oppositional and conduct problems?* Traditionally, irritability in young people has been seen as the hallmark of disruptive behaviour problems (conduct or oppositional disorders). However, by far the majority of irritability does not give rise to conduct or oppositional symptoms. The diagnostic criteria for ODD contain items (touchy, easily annoyed, and angry) that describe irritable mood, along with a number of other items that characterize behaviours (e.g. 'argues with adults' or 'disobeys'). Recent work suggests that children scoring high on the irritability items will have a different outcome from those scoring high on the items that characterize non-compliant and defiant behaviours. Young people with irritable mood are at increased risk of developing depressive or anxiety disorders, while those scoring high on the behaviour items are more likely to have ADHD or develop conduct problems. We suggest in Chapter 4 that irritability is a motivating mood for what has often been described as 'reactive aggression', but that it is less relevant in those with proactive, learned, or planned aggression, or in children with callous and unemotional traits.

♦ *Is irritability a manifestation of early-onset bipolar disorder?* The 'pediatric bipolar debate' arose in the United States following a vast increase in diagnosed cases of bipolar disorder in children as young as 4 years of age. Questions were raised about these diagnostic practices and their implications for young people (a vast increase in prescription rates for antipsychotic medication was observed at around the same time). Irritability seemed to be at the centre of this debate, in that it was considered by some researchers to be the most common and characteristic early manifestation of bipolar disorder. This view has been challenged on a number of grounds which are discussed in Chapter 10. It seems unlikely that typical bipolar disorder in children is very common, and irritability is certainly not specific to early bipolar disorder. Nevertheless clinicians, parents, and policy makers have until recently lacked an official description for children with severe irritability. The value of such a label—which is provided in DSM-5 but not in the World Health Organization's international classification of disorders—is discussed in Chapters 10 and 12.

♦ *Are there different pathways to irritability?* Clinicians often feel that the irritability in, say, a young boy with autism is somehow different from the irritability in an adolescent girl with depression. Certainly, the setting in which irritability manifests may differ across people. In autism, for example, irritability can occur as a result of sensory sensitivity or resistance to change (see Chapter 8), while in depression it can arise without a clear precipitant (during a period of sadness) or accompany self-deprecating thoughts (see Chapter 11). This may suggest that people arrive at irritability in different ways.

♦ *Does irritability affect treatment and how can it be treated itself?* Irritability is traditionally seen as a hindrance to treatment and as difficult to treat in its own right. Many clinicians would argue that in the presence of irritability it is difficult to treat, say, ADHD or depression. Yet the data suggest that treatment of ADHD, depression, mania, or other underlying problems often leads to considerable improvements in irritability; Chapter 14 presents options for treatment outside those coexistent diagnoses.

Chapter 2

Terminology

Definitions

Irritability can be defined as a state of proneness to anger. In this book we will take that definition as a starting point and try to extend or sharpen it as we move along. The roots of the word 'irritable' can be traced back to the Latin adjective 'irritabilis' meaning easily excited or easily enraged (Lewis and Short, 1879). It shares its roots with the Latin word 'ira', which is commonly translated into English as 'anger'. In Latin 'ira' seems to have had a fairly broad meaning. In the words of classicist William V. Harris (2002, p. 69):

> The term ira and its correlates had sometimes to do duty for mild anger, but the range included intense anger, for Cicero said, . . . that it is characteristic of the angry man to wish 'to inflict as much pain as possible' on his victim—which is too extreme for much modern anger.

The Latin roots for 'irritability' are reflected in the entries of modern dictionaries. The *Oxford English Dictionary* (OED, 2007), gives three related meanings:

- The familiar definition which refers to an emotional reaction: 'readily excited to anger or impatience, easily annoyed'.

- A second definition which refers to an overall increased sensitivity: '(of a thing) readily excited to action; highly responsive to stimulus; (of a bodily organ or part) excessively or abnormally sensitive'.

- A third definition comes closest to the biological one: 'capable of actively responding to a physical stimulus of some kind'.

According to *Chambers dictionary of etymology* (Barnhart, 1988), the meaning of annoyance or vexation for irritability was first recorded as late as 1703. Thus irritability is related to some kind of reactivity that may be emotionally unvalenced (e.g. the movement of a living organism in response to an electric stimulus) or valenced, as when describing someone who is easily angered.

It is important to note here that in these definitions irritability is described as a propensity. It is a propensity to become angry with relatively little provocation or with relatively high frequency, a meaning close to brittle. However, this definition as a propensity is not always evident in everyday usage. Consider the situation where someone who has just experienced hostility from another person turns to them saying: 'You are so irritable!' or 'Why are you so irritable?', or 'What made you so irritable?'. In these instances, 'irritable' refers to the hostile or angry reaction at that moment in time, rather than necessarily a person's propensity. This may be due to the fact that people form impressions about habitual responses or propensities (e.g. whether someone is irritable or not) even from single encounters. Also, anger—a word that is often taken as synonymous with irritability—is used as either a propensity ('an angry person', 'generally quite angry') or as descriptor of a current state, as in 'What made you so angry?'.

As we will be discussing, irritability is often used synonymously or nearly synonymously with a number of other words: we chose irritability rather than any of its synonyms or related words not least because 'irritability' is mostly used in official terminology referring to mood and anxiety disorders.

Irritability: mood, emotion, or temperament?

Irritability, in this book and in the wider psychiatric and psychological literature, is taken to refer to an emotionally coloured state. However, it is unclear whether irritability should be considered as a mood, an emotion, or a temperamental disposition.

The main distinction that is made between these three terms is duration: emotions are meant to last up to minutes, moods up to months (at least in pathological states), and temperaments years to decades (Ketter et al., 2003). Obviously, these distinctions are imprecise: what is the maximum number of minutes before an emotion can be called a mood, and how many months may a mood last until it is considered a temperament? Moreover, emotions, moods, and temperamental dispositions can be interdependent in their definitions. For example, if temperaments are predispositions to certain moods, then the only way of knowing about them would be through the repeated occurrence of certain moods. Furthermore, there seems an asymmetry between moods and emotions in the sense that only certain emotions can last for long enough to become moods; for example, it is hard to see how the relatively common emotion of surprise can become a mood. Conversely, it seems hard to translate the most commonly experienced moods into a concrete long-lasting emotion—it would seem that people's usual moods can be either neutral or contain a mixture of short-lasting usually mildly valenced states.

The question of the duration of emotionally valenced states has important practical implications. As will be discussed in more detail later, the duration of an emotional state can be crucial for classification and treatment decisions—as in distinctions between chronic and episodic irritability (Leibenluft et al., 2003).

In DSM-IV (APA, 2000), irritability was clearly referred to as a mood in the context of three disorders that are central to psychopathology: depression, dysthymia, and bipolar disorder. It is for this reason that we will refer to irritability as a mood in this book. We will return to the question of the relationship between irritability and constructs of temperament and personality, as well as its characterization as a mood, throughout this book.

Irritability and other closely related terms

Irritability is used to denote a propensity to reacting with anger. For most of this book we use the items 'touchy or easily annoyed', 'angry', and 'temper outbursts' to define the construct of irritability. The reasons for doing so will be explained, including precedents (Leibenluft et al., 2006) or near precedents (Angold et al., 1999; Brotman et al., 2006), and much of the book is devoted to the empirical scrutiny of this choice. It is, however, evident that in many situations that occur in everyday life the words 'irritability', 'anger', and 'temper outbursts' may be used interchangeably, along with words such as 'frustration', 'upset', or 'hostile'. Trying to draw firm semantic distinctions between such words is beyond the scope of this book and the reader is referred to publications highlighting the usefulness of such analyses (Ortony et al., 1990; Wierzbicka, 1999; Kagan, 2004). For the purposes of situating this book in the terminology used in the field of developmental psychiatry, we will briefly discuss in this section how irritability relates to other terms that are in common use. As discussed, irritability is commonly used to denote a high propensity to reacting with anger. A number of supraordinate terms can encompass irritability, most notably emotion dysregulation (see Fig. 2.1). Some such words in common use are 'emotion' (or 'emotional'), 'mood', or 'affect' (or 'affective') as adjectives with the word 'lability'. Often, instead of 'lability' the words 'instability' or 'dysregulation', or more rarely 'impulsivity' (Barkley et al., 2010), are used. Terms such as 'emotion lability' or 'mood lability' are supraordinate to irritability because they may refer to a propensity to manifest not only angry reactions but also other negative emotions (such as sadness) as well as positively valenced emotions (such as elation). Indeed, the term 'emotion (dys-)regulation' is commonly used in the context of discussions about adult bipolar disorder (Phillips et al., 2008) to denote fluctuations towards either positively or negatively valenced mood.

Similarly, 'mood lability' has been used to capture either negative or positive mood fluctuations in children and adolescents (Stringaris et al., 2009c).

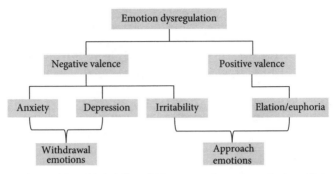

Fig. 2.1 The position of irritability within commonly used terminology. Note that irritability shares a negative valence with anxiety and depression, but is an approach emotion and is therefore linked to elation in mania.

However, a great part of the literature—particularly that concerning children and adolescents—uses such terms to denote negative affect. For example, the term mood dysregulation is used to describe the mood states of irritability and sadness (Leibenluft et al., 2003), and emotional lability is similarly used to denote negative affect, probably closest to irritability in Sobanski et al. (2010). Also emotion dysregulation is a term that is often used to describe negative affect (such as crying) but not elation in infants (Eisenberg, 2000). The three terms emotion (or emotional), mood, and affect (or affective) are used more or less interchangeably in this context. Similarly, the words stability, lability, and dysregulation are, in the context of the studies that are of primary interest to this book, used in ways that are nearly synonymous, denoting the fluctuation of emotion, mood, or affect. However, the term dysregulation has different connotations in the context of pathophysiological studies, where it usually implies a hypothesized aberrant function of a control instance (often a prefrontal cortical area; Leibenluft et al., 2007; Phillips et al., 2008) thought to underlie the fluctuation in emotions.

Chapter 3

Assessment of children with irritability

Is irritability a problem?

Irritability will often be the main reason for the referral of a child to a clinic. Parents and children may use a variety of terms to refer to the same problem. Box 3.1 lists some common ways of describing irritability.

There are other presentations, however, in which it is important to ask directly about problems of anger. Sometimes, young people and families present to a clinic with a problem that occurs *before* the feeling or other manifestation of irritability. Such events can vary from intense anxiety to problems with communication (see Johnny's case in Box 8.1), both of which may give rise to irritability. Similarly, the presenting complaint can be a problem that occurs *after* the manifestation of irritability. This is typically the case with children who end up having fights or being otherwise antisocial. In such cases it is easy for the clinician to overlook irritability.

Sometimes irritability is present and impairing, but is overshadowed by other problems such as disobedience and antisocial acts. An initial evaluation should include a screen for symptoms of irritability. At a busy clinic or in a primary-care setting this initial screen can be done using scales such as the Strengths and Difficulties Questionnaire (SDQ; Goodman, 1997) or the Child Behavior Checklist (CBCL; Achenbach, 1991), which enquire about psychopathology in general and include a few items on irritability.

Who reports irritability?

This will depend on characteristics of the clinical setting, such as the age range of the children referred or the area of psychopathology the clinic specializes in. Both parents and teachers will be good at noticing the behaviours that are characteristic of irritability, i.e. temper outbursts. Teachers are usually not as good at describing the intense distress that children feel as part of their irritability. Parents are usually better at recognizing the subjective suffering, the brooding, angry ruminations, and overall dysphoria that accompanies irritability. Young people themselves can be excellent at describing

Box 3.1 Commonly used terms to describe irritability

Angry
Bad-tempered
Cranky
Cross
Easily annoyed
Easily frustrated
Fractious
Grouchy
Grumpy
Mad (chiefly US)
Often annoyed
Pissed off
Quick-tempered
Short-tempered
Snappy
Tantrums
Touchy

their problems with anger: depending on their developmental level, children as young as 7 years of age can give very meaningful descriptions of things that go on before and after episodes of irritability and give a good account of their own feelings (see what Jack says in Box 7.1). Adolescents can be excellent at describing their feelings and give precise accounts of their problem (see Jane's case in Box 11.2). However, it is also not unusual for children to be either too embarrassed to give an account or simply to have a reduced awareness of their own symptoms. There are cases where only the child or only a parent describes irritability. Clinicians are used to some problems being described by some but not all informants. Importantly, there will be cases where nobody mentions irritability as a problem, but where anger, touchiness, and frustration are readily observable to clinicians.

Defining irritability

Because irritability can be a part of normal development, it is necessary to establish whether it is present at a clinically significant level. More specialist scales are available for research purposes, to guide the clinician, and to monitor progress (Stringaris et al., 2012a; Narrow et al., 2013). In the Appendix we provide such a scale that we have recently developed to capture irritability over the preceding 6 months. The gold standard is the clinical assessment, with interviews and observation.

As with every assessment it is important to establish that you and the patient mean the same thing when talking about irritability or anger. One of the best ways of achieving this is by asking the parents or young person to provide examples. Either the most recent or the most memorable (which is often the most severe) event with irritability is a useful anchoring point for the interview. Sometimes parents may respond by saying 'he's always like this' or may find it difficult to point out individual events. It is then worth asking the parents or young person to take you through a typical day. It is useful to use a whiteboard to note descriptors of irritable feelings or behaviours (such as those in Box 3.1) as you proceed with your assessment.

Intensity of temper outbursts

Chapter 4 considers tantrums in the framework of normal development. They need to be judged in the context of the child's developmental age. Was there a lot of provocation or do outbursts appear after only trivial annoyances? (Remember to check for social media confrontations or 'trolling'.) Are the tempers confined to angry facial expressions and grumbling? Do they include going red in the face, yelling, screaming, and stamping the feet? Do they go on to objects being thrown or broken? Do they impact on other people with verbal abuse, swearing, hitting, or kicking? Have they ever led to self-harm? Do they escalate rapidly through these levels? Are they distressing to the child? How long do they last? Do they resolve completely, or is there persisting vindictiveness or spitefulness towards the objects of the tantrum?

Frequency and chronicity

Clinicians will want to know whether irritability occurs as discrete episodes, for example a period of a week of extreme irritability, or as something chronic, that is, a set of feelings and behaviours that have been typical of the young person for a considerable period of time. Drawing a time line—perhaps on a board or a large sheet of paper in the consulting room—can be quite helpful.

Fig. 3.1 shows two examples that highlight the distinction between discrete and chronic states. The solid line describes the irritability of an 8-year-old boy, Johnny, brought to you by his parents because of persistent irritable mood (see Box 8.1) and several temper outbursts per day. He was given a diagnosis of ODD, but in the new DSM-5 he would qualify for disruptive

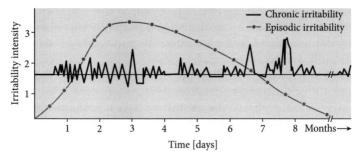

Fig. 3.1 Time patterns in irritability. The dashed line depicts the episodic irritability of a young person with mania who was treated early on (at about day 3) and who also had a number of other manic symptoms. The solid line shows the persistent grumpy mood (straight line that persists throughout) and the superimposed tantrums (shown as spikes); these are the characteristic elements of chronic irritability, for example as defined in severe mood dysregulation and disruptive mood dysregulation disorder.

mood dysregulation disorder (DMDD; see Chapter 12). The dashed line in Fig. 3.1 depicts the irritability of a girl, Jane, who has recently experienced a short-lived (a week's duration) episode of extreme irritability for the first time in her life (see Box 11.2). She also experienced other symptoms of mania during this time, such as disinhibition, hypersexuality, overspending, and a reduced need for sleep. As will be discussed, this distinction is of great diagnostic value in distinguishing classical bipolar disorder from the more common manifestation of chronic irritability.

Enduring feelings of anger can be harder to elicit. When a child is old enough, their description of their feelings in interview (or by an impersonal self-report, e.g. on screen) will be the best guide. It will allow discrimination between miserable and angry thoughts, observation of sadness when particular topics are touched on, and listening to angry ruminations. If this is not practical, because the child is not yet articulate enough, or trusting enough, to give a subjective account, then ratings by adults who know the child well may be sufficient. One should, however, be careful not to accept inferential ratings—stick to recollections of what the child has said or done.

Context and antecedents

It is not uncommon for irritability to manifest in particular circumstances only, such as when a person is reminded of certain events (see Chapter 11) or confronted with particular challenges (see Chapter 8). However, irritability can be pervasive, particularly in severe cases occurring at home, at school, or during leisure with friends. Regardless of where irritability mostly manifests, it is important to search for what may have triggered it. Useful questions to ask are: what time of the day is the irritability worst, what is the main activity of the young person at the time, and does the irritability coincide with particular changes? In Jack's case (Box 7.1), irritability was at its worst later in the day on days when he was attending school. This was when his ADHD medication was wearing off and he improved dramatically with a small addition of short-acting methylphenidate. In Jane's case (Box 11.2, Chapter 11), ruminations and thoughts of self-reproach are strongest before she snaps at her mother or boyfriend. Parents or patients should be asked to keep a diary—usually in the form of a chart—detailing irritable mood and the actions, thoughts, or other events that precede it. Particular foods are often incriminated by parents, and a food diary can help them to test their hypothesis.

The family and school context may also be a long-term issue. Clinicians should consider whether the anger may be accounted for by a predictable response to stresses under which the child is living. For example, it is common for children receiving harsh physical punishment to develop high levels of resentment and even aggression to others (see Chapter 4). Furthermore, underachievement at school—and even more being blamed for it—may fuel an angry rejection of the situation and a sentiment that the world is unfair.

Care should be taken not to imply blame when questioning parents about these issues. If the parents have become angry it may be because they have been strongly provoked by mental disturbance in their child. Whether parental hostility is reactive and expected or derives from their own mental state, it can still be a target for planning treatment.

Home observation is a sensitive, but expensive, means of assessing the antecedents and consequences of irritability. Prolonged and repeated observations may well be needed because of the distorting effect of an observer in the situation. Diary keeping and recording on tablets or smartphones may be more realistic approaches.

Consequences

There are both immediate and longer-term consequences to consider. The impact may be on other members of the family as well as the young person—Who is most distressed? According to whom?

What is the situation at school? Is the child being victimized, or are his/her angry reactions causing ostracism or revenge attacks? Are there many fights? Are other children suffering—from abuse, face-to-face or via social media, or from violence?

How have other people reacted? This is best investigated by asking for memories of concrete instances. Has a temper outburst secured benefit for the child, for example by achieving escape from a frustrating situation or gaining the initial purpose of a tantrum? Rewards may not be immediately obvious, and the effect of social attention can be gratifying: how much fuss was there?

Was the child expected to 'make up' to anyone who was the object of the temper? Was there any punishment, and if so what form did it take? Were the people giving punishment angry themselves and did a cycle of hostile coercion develop? Is there a general climate of hostility in the family?

Modifiability

Was the child able to control the temper themself? Or was the temper soothed by others? Distraction to other activities, physical cuddling, swiftly allowing the child to gain the desired object, and isolation are all commonly used methods (see Chapter 4): how much had to be employed and how quickly did it work? It is also helpful to get an idea about how much agreement there is between family members on the reactions to be adopted and about the extent to which carers have modified their responses in the light of their consequences. This may give useful leads on the advice that can be given and the opportunities for parental training on behavioural modification.

Instruments

Screening for irritability can be kept very simple without instruments. Any of the synonyms in Box 3.1 can be used to screen for irritability; you can then ask about duration, frequency, and consequences. You can save time by using a screening instrument such as the Affective Reactivity Index (ARI, see Appendix), and this will also allow you to quantify levels of irritability and the impairment that results from it.

Drawing a timeline on a piece of paper or a whiteboard to distinguish between chronic and episodic irritability can help you to get a better overview of the duration and frequency of tantrums. Ask your patient or his/her parent(s) to keep diaries recording their mood. This will be a helpful way to map out antecedents and consequences. It will also be helpful when you plan the child's treatment (Stringaris et al., 2010).

Is the irritability part of a complex disorder?

Irritability often coexists with other disorders, and the extent to which this is the case may dominate treatment planning. Coexisting conditions such as

ADHD, depression, and bipolar disorder may have specific treatments that should be employed at an early stage, and the context of those specific conditions will be described separately in Chapters 7, 11, and 10, respectively. Chapter 14 will then take up their differential diagnosis and the general management of irritability.

The initial stages of clinical contact will end with the formulation of a therapeutic plan, which must be conveyed in suitable terms to the child and the responsible adults, and setting up systems for the monitoring of the response to intervention.

Chapter 4

The development of anger

Anger is a normal emotion. Like other emotions, it has elements of subjective feeling states, overt behaviour of various kinds, and bodily changes. Charles Darwin, in his classic work *The expression of the emotions in man and animals*, published in 1872, regarded anger as one of the basic emotions, present from an early stage of development. Darwin considered anger to be an adaptive function evoked when there was an obstacle to attaining a goal, and designed to overcome it (Barrett, 2011).

There are several lines for the development of anger during childhood and adolescence: the intensity and frequency of occurrence of the mood, the environmental features that evoke it, its expression in behaviour, its effect on and modification by other people, and the extent to which the young person controls it. The ability to recognize emotions in oneself and others is a developing function which modifies the other lines of development. Anger can be either functional or dysfunctional, according to context, but it is very often disapproved of.

Infancy

Expression of anger

Infants do not, of course, express their feelings in words, but they convey them clearly with their bodies. Parents recognize the flushed face, the scowl, and the vocalizations. Researchers such as Izard have developed several coding systems for facial movements (Izard et al., 1995) that allow a reliable recognition and even quantification of the mood state. On this basis it is possible to say that by the age of 2 to 3 months babies are reacting to frustration or violation of expectancy, and by the age of 5 to 6 months that anger is indeed elicited by the same situations. If, for instance, spontaneous hand movements are checked by an adult's restraint, or if a piece of food is removed from a child when it is hungry and expecting to eat, then the combination of the situation and facial expression imply that anger is a good way of describing the child's reactions. A sudden absence of parental responsiveness (the 'still-face' situation) is also used experimentally to elicit similar reactions (Adamson et al., 2003). Soothing and comforting by the parent is the beginning of emotional control.

Frustration tends to elicit both anger and sadness, and infants differ in the extent to which they show these two reactions. In a study by Michael Lewis and colleagues, sadness, not anger, was associated with a significant increase in cortisol measured in saliva (Lewis et al., 2005). This can be seen as a stress response. Anger is associated more with attempts to overcome the obstacle, and in this situation at least it is a more positive reaction than sadness.

Perception of anger

Infants can discriminate between the emotions, as expressed by other people, from an early stage of development. When they are shown pictures of angry, joyful, and neutral faces they look at the representations of anger for shorter periods than they do for those of joy; this can be observed from as early as 4 months of age (LaBarbera et al., 1976).

By the age of 12 months one can expect children to express and recognize anger in a social context. They are referencing their parents' reactions to them and others, and may react to their parents' anger with anger themselves. Bandura's experimental work (Bandura, 1973) stressed children's imitation of the social interactions they saw and heard; more naturalistic observational studies have indicated that the emotional response is important (see Box 4.1).

Box 4.1 A study of children's emotional responses

Mark Cummings and colleagues (Cummings et al., 1981) studied 24 children aged between 10 and 20 months and their reactions to both natural and simulated episodes of both angry and affectionate interactions between other people. The children's mothers were trained as observers, and their ratings of children's behaviour were reliable.

When there had been an angry episode in the family—for instance between the mother and the father—then the children reacted, most often with distress and crying but quite often with angry behaviours such as verbal scolding, or pushing or hitting the people involved, or unfocused yelling. They did not usually imitate the aggression directly, but showed the emotion appropriate to it.

By contrast, their reaction to spontaneous episodes of affection was much more likely to be one of pleasure. When they did react with a behaviour such as pushing, it tended to be a jealous attempt to win affection for themselves, and not to be accompanied by distress.

Children who were exposed to higher levels of aggression at home were more likely to react to anger with anger.

Regulation of anger

In the first months of life the expression of emotions generally, and of anger in particular, comes to be modified by the ability of caregivers to soothe and comfort and infants' growing capacity to modify their own state.

Parental soothing is guided by the reaction of the infant. As time goes by, it includes physical comfort and rocking, distraction, and modelling by the parent. Modelling may involve the parent displaying a moderate level of comparable distress—less than that of the child, of course—and then reducing it. Verbal intervention can be soothing in itself, and can also convey meaning and a labelling of the mood state: 'I know, you're all cross, never mind'.

There is also the start of emotional regulation by children themselves, as voluntary actions increasingly enter their repertoire. They may well be beginning to comfort themselves, for instance with thumb-sucking; sometimes repetitive activities such as head-banging start with a self-regulating function but then become a problem in their own right. As development proceeds, attentional control becomes available as a means of emotional regulation. Observers can see a child looking, or moving, away from frustrating stimuli. This is typical of frustrating situations, but it contrasts with reactions in situations arousing fear (when attention is often strongly focused on a scary object and the related movement is towards safety). Typically, too, attentional control is only used, or only effective, when the level of arousal is relatively low; an intense fury is not managed in this way (or has already exceeded any such attempt).

Researchers have taken up the question of whether these behaviours by the infant can truly be seen as self-regulation. (They might, for example, be simply a concomitant of the emotion.) The concept of regulation (see Chapter 2) includes the idea of adaptive behaviours with the function and effect of modifying the intensity, quality, and frequency of emotional expression. One way of testing this is whether the behaviour does indeed have the effect of reducing the direct expression of the emotion. For instance, Buss and Goldsmith (1998) activated negative emotions in children aged 6, 12, or 18 months. To elicit anger they restrained the young children's arms or prevented them from reaching to an attractive toy. The supposedly self-regulating behaviours were activities such as directing gaze away from the frustration, getting closer to the caregiver, or sucking parts of their bodies. Emotional intensity was recorded separately, and it showed that anger levels (but not levels of fear) were reduced after the attempts at regulation.

Another way of testing whether some behaviours are indeed regulatory rather than simple emotional expressions is to compare how different children relate to emotional intensity. For instance, Calkins et al. (2002) contrasted infants at 6 months of age who were easily frustrated (according to parental report) with those who were less frustratable: the former used less self-regulation (such as looking away) and more overt emotional behaviour—including bigger changes in heart rate variability.

Preschool

During the preschool period, i.e. around the ages of 2 to 5 years, there is an increasing complexity in both the expression and control of anger (see Box 4.2). Children's increasing competence in cognition, language, and motor skills allows them to use more methods of controlling their emotions. They use self-soothing less, and complex interactions with people more (Diener et al., 1999). Parental regulation is still important: studies of parental interaction with toddlers and preschoolers indicate that mutual regulation of emotion is the key mode of interaction (Cole et al., 2003). Effortful inhibitory self-control becomes possible; and indeed the extent to which toddlers check themselves is predicted by the early quality of dyadic emotion regulation between the parent and child in infancy (Feldman et al., 1999).

Overt and covert anger

The typical overt expression of anger is the tantrum. In a survey by Wakschlag et al. (2012) temper tantrums were very common in children: 83.7% of 3–5-year-olds had had one in the course of the previous month (indeed, 8.6% had had daily tantrums). Yelling (and, later, abuse), limb-shaking (and, later, physical attack), and autonomic changes (flushing, tachycardia) occur in an episode—typically lasting up to a minute. The length, however, is very variable because much depends on parental skill in redirecting the child's

Box 4.2 A study of influences on the expression of anger

Richard Fabes and Nancy Eisenberg (1992) studied preschool children (mean age 55 months) and observed how they reacted to provocation. Several influences on emotional expression were seen:

- ◆ Children who were popular and made good relationships with other children had also acquired a variety of ways of coping actively with provoking situations. They found responses that reduced conflict.
- ◆ Girls tended to be more effectively assertive than boys, while boys were more likely to respond with physical signs of anger.

focus, but up to 15 minutes is not unusual. Tantrums comprise both anger and distress. The anger typically starts first, but can be followed by crying and comfort-seeking (Potegal et al., 2003). They are both individual passions and social events. Usually there is a short pause for rest during the course of one, and some referencing of others, in looking for a reaction.

Skilled parents will find that they can note early when anger is developing, judge its likely intensity, and either distract the child or remove the provocation. Once a tantrum has developed, however, even experienced parents may find it hard to modify and will often separate themselves from a screaming child. During a tantrum there is often a very limited connection with other people. The details of it are often forgotten afterwards. This has two clinical consequences: a rage can be misinterpreted as a seizure (see Chapter 13), and it is pointless to reason during a tantrum. Rather (and see Chapter 14), a tantrum is often followed later by a period of remorse during which a child can often appreciate explanations and suggestions for the future.

The persistence and frequency of tantrums is influenced by whether they succeed in influencing other people, the form of parental discipline, the emotional availability of parent(s), the extent to which discipline is perceived by the child as unfair, the models of anger the child sees, and, sometimes, even by overt encouragement by parents in conflict with each other. Inhibitory control is also developing at this age, and the child's ability to hold back immediate overt responses will play a part.

Covert anger

Covert and prolonged anger is linked to children's perception and appraisal of how they are treated. Strong feelings of resentment can be linked to feeling unfairly dealt with, or coerced or humiliated. It can be exacerbated by a sense of helplessness, or of conflicting rules that make it impossible to be correct. Misconceptions can arise; for example, perception of unavoidable misfortune as being maliciously intended or of a parent as being hostile or neglectful when, in fact, this represents misrepresentation by the other parent (parental alienation).

During this period of life, children begin to describe their states verbally ('Eddie cross') and to link their feelings to their external causes. They understand the consequences better and acquire the ability to use the behaviours of anger not only to express irritation but to control other people. They learn to talk with their caregivers about what makes them cross and how that affects other people. They increasingly develop the capacity to describe other people's emotions (typically, positive emotions such as happiness before negative ones such as anger). Constructive coping with anger-provoking situations becomes possible: they develop, for example, skills in compromise with other children when their interests conflict. The greater the use of attentional control and constructive coping, and the less the emotional intensity of anger, the less likely children are to use abusive language or to run away from the situation (Eisenberg et al., 1994).

School age and adolescence

After the transition into school, from around the age of 5, increasing sophistication lets young people mask their anger, and learn what it can achieve and what the costs are (especially in the reactions of other children). They can attend to and appraise situations that will potentially arouse anger. The increased ability of children to monitor their own emotional state allows early recognition that they are losing their temper, and at that early stage decision-making about how to respond becomes feasible. They also come to understand the rules and context—for instance, that what is acceptable if you are a boy may be different from that for a girl.

There is an increasing gap between boys and girls in their expression of physical aggression, due largely to a minority of boys who deploy aggression at high rates (Hay et al., 2011). This is not paralleled by a major gender difference in the experience of anger (unlike the case for depression). Stringaris et al. (2012b) reported that scores on an irritability scale were significantly higher in girls than in boys (means of 2.27 versus 1.86, respectively); by contrast scores on the headstrong/hurtful behaviour scale were significantly higher in boys than in girls (means of 1.84 versus 1.38). The male vulnerability to developmental problems, the early development of prosocial skills in girls, and cultural expectations based on gender are probably all involved.

Peer relationships become increasingly differentiated. Friendship groups, gender roles, and hierarchies of dominance and popularity become established. Some children are becoming rejected by their peers, and experience loneliness, bullying, and victimization. These are not only causes of frustration and anger, but can be consequences of their own abusive anger. A cycle of problems with peers and personal maladjustment can then appear.

Covert, long-term changes of affect may not be evident to others, but exist as subjective hostility—that can then influence the extent to which the children may indulge revenge or destructive hatred. For some children, a ready and forceful recourse to anger and/or aggression becomes attractive—not only by getting them what they want, but also as an expression of power and status. For others, the experience of anger is unpleasant and aversive and they try to suppress it.

Adulthood

By early adult life, Averill's surveys (Averill, 1982) indicated a usual frequency of one or two episodes of anger a week, but with only one in ten of them leading to aggression. In adulthood there are more and more ways in which to influence other people short of physical or verbal violence. Individual differences in the use of effortful control are associated with differences in angry reactivity (Wilkowski et al., 2008). Automatic hostile interpretations about the behaviour of other people may have become ingrained, and ruminative attention to the wrongs one has experienced may exacerbate pervasive feelings of anger. Both personal makeup and learned responses from childhood remain influential: adult antisocial behaviour and adult depression are both predicted by early childhood anger (Caspi et al., 1996).

There is rather little difference between the genders in self-reports of anger/hostility. The differences, which are not spectacular, come from what elicits anger (more likely to be in the context of close personal relationships for females) and how it is expressed (with males more likely to hit and females to use words or to cry) (Averill, 1982).

Anger and aggression

Though anger and aggression are associated with each other from the first months of life, as soon as children have the physical competence to display aggression they are not the same thing.

Aggression in development can be classified in various ways. Animal researchers distinguish predatory and defensive types. Many of the human distinctions—reflected in bold type in Box 4.3—relate to the distinction between a 'hot' form of aggression driven by anger and a 'cold' form reflecting learned behaviour and decision-making.

Box 4.3 Classification of aggression

Competitive versus **Impulsive**
Instrumental versus **Hostile**
Proactive versus **Reactive**
Unemotional versus **Affective**
Covert versus **Overt**
Direct versus Indirect
Physical versus Verbal

Physiological changes during anger include an elevated heart rate and the cortisol response, as described by Scarpa and Raine (1997). These occur in response to most kinds of stress, and do not differentiate anger from other states of emotional arousal. Individuals who are unusually prone to the emotional–hostile–impulsive forms of aggression tend to react strongly to stimuli with increases in skin conductance and heart rate. Chronic states of anger, however, may be associated with blunted cortisol and heart rate responses.

Individual differences

In all these lines of development there is a great deal of individual variation. Some of it derives from the child's own temperament and some of it comes from the ways in which he or she is treated.

Genetic influences

Anger is heritable from an early age. Gagne and Hill Goldsmith (2011) studied more than 700 children, who were either monozygotic or dizygotic twins, on the basis of parental ratings of both anger and inhibitory control. As would be expected from the developmental considerations highlighted, high anger tended to correlate with low inhibitory control. The information from parental ratings confirmed earlier findings that genetic influences were significant for anger at both 12 and 36 months of age (accounting for about 72% and 45%, respectively, of the variance in scores) and for inhibitory control at 36 months (63%).

These researchers were also able to apply laboratory assessments—tests such as eliciting anger by gentle restraint and inhibitory control by having to wait for a few seconds before eating a chosen snack or selecting just one toy from a range of several. These gave partial support, with lower but still significant heritability for anger at 12 months (38%) and 36 months (32%). There was, however little correlation between the 12- and 36-month tests of anger; and the main influences on inhibitory control came from the shared and non-shared environment with scant evidence for any genetic factors.

In the kindergarten and early school years there is still evidence of modest heritability. Deater-Deckard et al. (2007) report a twin study in 4–8-year-olds, with 105 pairs of monozygotic twins and 154 pairs of same-sex dizygotic twins. Anger/frustration, observed by researchers during home visits, showed a heritability around 30%, with rather larger influences from the non-shared environment. This study also measured persistence as an index of self-control requiring effort. This had a similar level of heritability; and in addition they were able to show that persistence and anger/frustration were both linked to oppositional behaviour—but independently.

In adolescence, too, genetic influences play a part. Aebi et al. (2012) compared the different levels of similarity between monozygotic and dizygotic twins who reported their own irritability. About 30% of the inter-individual variation was due to genetic factors, and nearly all the rest was due to influences of the non-shared environment (i.e. the environmental influences that do not impact on both twins to the same degree). Headstrong/hurtful behaviour had a slightly higher heritability estimate—about 45%—but here too the non-shared environment played a strong role. This is in keeping with studies in adult samples (Coccaro et al., 1997).

Another finding emerging from a twin/sibling study by Stringaris et al. (2012b) study was that the overlap between irritability and depression was due to shared genetic effects. Irritability and depression differed from each other as a result of specific environmental effects.

Psychosocial influences

Non-shared environmental influences seem to be important from the twin studies, more so than those that operate across all the children in a family. (Shared environment does, however, play a part in determining individual differences in aggression and other antisocial behaviours.) Some of the main factors that distinguish one child from others in the family are connected with parenting.

Parental reactions are occasionally counter-productive. A young child who is consistently put into isolation because of a temper may not learn how to reduce anger in ways other than exhaustion. Children who do not understand why people are angry with them, or why their needs are not being met, may develop a long-lasting sense of resentment. A child whose parents match anger with anger may react with increasing intensity of irritabililty. An abused child may react with a profound and enduring hostility, not only to the abusers but to the generality of the adult world.

These interpersonal processes have been most studied for the overt behaviours of aggression rather than the subjective emotional concomitants (see Box 4.4).

Harshness of discipline, and the use of physical punishment by parents, are reliably associated with aggressive behaviour by the offspring. Within the ordinary range, this represents an interaction between the environment in which the child grows up and the genetic constitution of the child. For instance, one version of the monoamine oxidase A gene (*MAOA*), which codes for a protein that affects the level of neurotransmitters in the brain, influences whether children exposed to a harsh environment become aggressive themselves (Kim-Cohen et al., 2006). By contrast, the extreme level of hostility that constitutes physical abuse appears to overwhelm the innate

Box 4.4 The birthday party

Dale Hay and her colleagues (Hay et al., 2011) used simulated birthday parties to observe the levels of aggression shown by 271 infants aged 12 months. High levels of aggression were predicted by several factors, notably:

- children's levels of anger as rated by parents
- maternal depression during pregnancy
- history of conduct problems in the mother.

These influences are also associations of violence in later development, so the links arise early.

disposition of the child to react; children exposed in this way are very likely to become aggressive, whatever their genetic predisposition.

Individual differences in aggression tend to persist over time; instrumental aggression waxes or wanes according to its effectiveness in achieving the individual's goals. Prosocial emotions—such as one's response to the distress of others—work to reduce aggressive behaviour. Anxiety about others' reactions moderates any tendencies to be cruel, while language development increases the range of opportunities to convey one's feelings without physical contact.

Cultural differences

There can also be differences between children from different cultural backgrounds. Culture can affect all the lines of development considered here. The situations provoking anger, the way that those situations are thought of in the culture, children's understanding of the situations, their perceptions of anger in others, their expression of anger in behaviour, feelings, and bodily reactions, and the control of emotional expression by expectations and child-rearing practices can all differ between different cultures (Mesquita and Frijda, 1992). Their influence should not be discounted because of the apparent lack of shared environmental influences from twin studies conducted in single cultures. The influence of ethnically or religiously influenced practices will often be on the reactions of families, schools, and society to individual differences expressed by the children.

Research has often approached these influences by comparisons between children in different ethnic groups. It is unwise to summarize a culture, but Japan and the United States are often contrasted for the collectivist atmosphere of the former, with shame playing a valued role in making for conformity; and the individualist atmosphere of the latter, with a valued emphasis on independence and emotional expressiveness.

Zahn-Waxler et al. (1996) found that young Japanese children were less prone than American children to aggression and displays of anger. On the other hand, at another time and using different means of eliciting emotional expression, Bear et al. (2009) found that Japanese children followed their predictions in expressing more shame and guilt—but confounded them by showing (slightly) more anger than their American counterparts. (It was nevertheless the case that more guilt was associated with less blaming and less anger within the Japanese group.) Chinese children asked to describe responses to ambiguous situations gave more angry responses than did Americans, especially when the stories involved frustrations from adults rather than peers (Borke et al., 1972).

It is one thing to note differences between nations but quite another to disentangle the multiple and confounded processes involved. Cultural influences are partly exerted through the microcultures of families. For example, a study in rural Nepal contrasted two communities—Tamang and Brahman—that were similar in demographics and collectivist atmosphere but different in attitudes (Cole et al., 2006). Tamang caregivers usually responded to children's anger with rebukes and teasing, and regarded anger as dysfunctional. Brahman caregivers, by comparison, were more likely to reason with, or coax, an angry child. This could well have been related to the tendency for Tamang children to describe feelings of shame in hypothetical conflict situations but for Brahman children to describe control of anger.

Lessons for clinicians are to be sensitive to cultural and religious beliefs and attitudes, but not to stereotype. They should not, for instance, automatically assume that a very irritable Japanese child is more deviant, or more severely affected by disorder, than an equivalent child from a dominant Western culture. Rather, they should be prepared to listen to and understand the values presented by a family, their reactions to and conversations about anger, and the models that the parents present to children about the expression of anger and its acceptability.

Normal and abnormal irritability

The presence of wide individual variation in children in their irritability raises a major issue of what level should be seen as 'abnormal'. This is a complex judgement. Wakschlag et al. (2007) set out some normative considerations derived from the distinction between typically developing children in preschool and those who were categorized as disruptive. The disruptive children's tempers were more likely to be intense and uncontrolled (see Box 4.5).

The severity, intensity and quality of tempers correlate with their frequency. Indeed, in a study of 1516 children aged between 3 and 5 years the features of tantrums reported by mothers on a detailed questionnaire could be ordered statistically into a single continuum of severity along which children varied (Wakschlag et al., 2012).

One study of 6- and 7-year-old children drawn from the general population asked parents for details of how many tempers they had in a week, and at what level of intensity they had been shown (Taylor et al., 1991). There was no clear cut-off for the link with oppositional/defiant problems. Of those children identified by parent and teacher questionnaires as showing conduct problems, 9/40 had a temper outburst on at least 3 days in the week; but this was only slightly more than the equivalent figure for those who were not so rated (6/41). The clinical judgement is not governed only by the intensity and frequency of tempers. It should include their quality and controllability, together with the extent to which they are out of keeping with any provocation or with the developmental age of the child, and whether they are causing harm—either to the child or other people.

It follows from this account that there are many ways in which the influences normally operating to shape the expression of anger can produce extreme levels of irritability. The levels of frustration to which children are exposed, the extent to which they have been shown how to recognize their anger and in what ways to express it, the extent to which the expression of

Box 4.5 Characteristics of tempers in disruptive versus typical children

In an observational study of preschool children, involving 50 minutes of play and different tasks, Lauren Wakschlag and colleagues (Wakschlag et al., 2012) found that the tempers of the disruptive children were more likely to be:

♦ Intense: loud, active, strong and forceful movements.

♦ Easily elicited: could occur after only slight provocation.

♦ Progressive: rapidly escalating to a crescendo.

♦ Pervasive: observed during several different tasks.

♦ Persistent: slow to recover and needing adult attention to resolve.

anger is tolerated in their milieu, and the reactions of other children and adults can all have substantial effects and interact with children's own constitutions. There are also individual differences in exposure to influences from the physical environment.

In clinical practice it is not always possible to understand the details of the history. Nevertheless the observation of current interactions with the people or situations to whom/to which their anger is directed can give useful clues about the processes that might be modified.

These multiple influences give rise to a continuum of severity, and the point at which it becomes impairing for the individual, or intolerable to others, will depend very much upon the context in which it occurs. Some aspects of treatment (see Chapter 14) depend upon encouraging the positive aspects of the processes promoting regulation referred to here. Often, however, unacceptable levels of irritability occur in the specific context of a psychiatric disorder; and succeeding chapters will consider them separately.

Chapter 5

Prevalence, comorbidity, and course across development

How common is irritability?

The answer to the question 'How common is irritability?' depends on what one considers to be the point beyond which irritability becomes relevant either clinically or in some other important way (e.g. because it predicts some important future outcome). A common practice in psychiatry is to generate a category for a disorder or a syndrome, for example one does or doesn't have major depressive disorder. This decision is based on pre-conceived—often described as a priori—notions of what is or might be relevant. The most prominent example of such an approach for irritability has been the category of severe mood dysregulation (SMD). This label has been used to capture children with severe irritability (discussed in Chapter 10) and the new DSM-5 diagnosis of disruptive mood dysregulation disorder (DMDD; discussed in Chapter 12). The other approach is to regard irritability as something that can be measured on a scale, perhaps similar to temperature or blood pressure. This is commonly termed a dimensional approach, and researchers often try to establish a threshold along such a scale. Many studies have used irritability scales to investigate its long-term outcomes, providing useful insights; however, no study has produced specific thresholds. Therefore, the discussion in this chapter on how common irritability is will be based on a priori categories.

US findings: prevalence of severe mood dysregulation

About 3% of children aged between 9 and 19 years had at some point in their lives met criteria for SMD (Brotman et al., 2006). If SMD were a disorder, it would have to be considered an uncommon one compared with other disorders: the cumulative prevalence of depression in the same cohort was 9.5%, of anxiety 9.9%, of ODD 11.3%, and of conduct disorder 9.0%. As noted, prevalence depends on definition. SMD requires the presence of both irritable mood for at least half of the day on most days and tantrums occurring on top of this, for a period of 12 months (see Box 10.1 and Chapter 10 for a detailed description of SMD). The rates were similar for the new category of Disruptive Mood Dysregulation Disorder (DMDD, see chapter 12) (Copeland et al., 2013), with higher rates occurring in young children.

UK findings: the Isle of Wight

Adolescents and parents interviewed as part of the Isle of Wight study (Pickles et al., 2010) were also asked about irritability. The responses were rated for frequency, severity, and duration of irritability, and these were coded as present if they were deemed to be significant on that basis. Approximately 19.1% of boys and 23.9% of girls were rated as displaying significant irritability. As will be explained later, irritability was a significant predictor of later outcomes in this sample.

UK findings: mood lability in a community sample

While there are no studies assessing the prevalence of SMD in other parts of the world, a community study on mood lability may give us some clues about it. As mentioned in Chapter 2, mood lability is one of the terms used to describe changes in mood that include irritability. When people are asked about mood lability, they often seem to refer to irritable mood as evidenced by the high correlation between the two constructs. In a study by Stringaris et al. (2009c), 6.1% of young people (aged 11–19) self-reported as having a lot of mood lability, and 5.5% of parents reported that their children (age range 8–19 years) suffered from a lot of mood lability. One of the striking findings of this study was that there was not much overlap between parental reporting of mood lability and children's views of their own mood lability. However, as we will see later, mood lability—no matter by whom it is reported—seems to carry clinical significance in its own right.

How common are tantrums?

Temper tantrums are a characteristic symptom of irritability, as discussed in Chapter 2. Also, as discussed in Chapter 4, tantrums have been studied across development and questions remain about how common they are at different developmental stages. A recent study (Wakschlag et al., 2010) shows that, as one would expect, temper tantrums are very common in young children, occurring in as many as 83.7% of 3–5-year-olds at some point over the past month. However, only 8.6% of those children had daily tantrums. Moreover, tantrums that came out of the blue or led to extreme behaviours, such as kicking or screaming, were much rarer.

Associations of irritability

Is irritability associated with any other problems, such as other psychiatric disorders, and are children with irritability more likely to suffer from problems with psychosocial adjustment? More importantly, do such associations last across time; for example, are children with irritability more likely than others to have a psychiatric disorder? Answering these questions is crucial in order to understand whether irritability is something innocuous or not.

To summarize the main points. Children with irritability are:

- more likely to have one or more of a range of psychiatric disorders, including emotional (e.g. depression) and behavioural (e.g. ADHD) disorders when seen in clinics or the community;
- at increased risk for future emotional problems, particularly depression, dysthymia, and generalized anxiety and probably suicidality;
- more likely to show poor social adjustment that is over and above what could be explained by psychopathology.

Irritability is associated with a range of psychiatric disorders

In a large UK community sample (Stringaris et al., 2009d), irritability—defined using a scale made up of the items of tantrums, anger, and touchiness—was associated with a wide range of disorders cross-sectionally. When looked at on its own, irritability was related to ADHD and disruptive and emotional disorders. The association was more specific for emotional disorders once the dimensions of oppositional behaviour other than irritability were controlled for (see Chapter 9).

Using the mood lability rather than the irritability construct in the same study showed a similarly wide association with a number of psychiatric disorders, by both parent and self-report (Stringaris et al., 2009c). One of the particularly striking findings of that study was that mood lability was strongly associated with *comorbidity*, i.e. the overlap between two or more disorders—especially the overlap between emotional and behavioural disorders.

Irritability is a predictor of emotional problems

A series of studies conducted in different parts of the world have shown that irritability is more strongly related to later emotional problems rather than antisocial outcomes.

In the UK, the longitudinal follow-up of the study by Stringaris et al. (2009b) showed that irritability was a significantly stronger predictor of distress disorders—a combination category of depression and generalized anxiety—than of conduct problems 3 years later. Also, the prediction to 'distress disorders' was significantly stronger than that to so-called 'fear disorders', a category encompassing phobias and post-traumatic stress disorder (PTSD).

In the United States, the first study to show that irritability was a fairly specific predictor of depression was the Children in the Community study (Leibenluft et al., 2006; Stringaris et al., 2009a). In this study, children and adolescents were followed up at various time points as they were moving through adolescence into mid adulthood. The 10- and 20-year follow-ups of the study both showed that irritability was a predictor of depression. The relationship was fairly strong: in the 20-year follow-up, irritability predicted depression, dysthymia, and generalized anxiety with an odds ratio of two, meaning that for every increase in one standard deviation of the irritability scale there was a doubling of the risk for depressive disorders. Moreover, irritability remained a predictor of future depressive disorders and generalized anxiety once other childhood psychiatric disorders present at baseline had been taken into account. Conversely, the prediction to other disorders, including phobias, personality disorders, and bipolar disorder, was non-significant.

The findings were similar in other studies investigating the outcomes of irritability. The findings do not seem to be specific to the UK. A recent investigation using a large Brazilian sample found that irritability was associated with depressive disorders, rather than antisocial behaviours (Krieger et al., 2013).

In another UK community study of adolescent outcomes, it was found that irritability predicted specifically to depression over antisocial outcomes. An important aspect of this study was that irritability was reported by the adolescents themselves rather than their parents or teachers (Stringaris et al., 2012b). Similar findings have been found in other studies from the United States (Burke, 2012).

Irritability is a predictor of social role impairment

We have seen that young people with irritability are at an increased risk for psychiatric disorders. In addition, they are also at an increased risk for social impairment. In the DMDD study by Copeland et al. (2013, also see chapter 12), young people with irritability were more likely to have problems in their relationships with their parents and siblings, be suspended from school, and be in trouble with the law. In the UK study, children with mood lability suffered impairment in their family lives and their relationships with peers as well as at school, and at a significantly higher rate than did children without mood lability

(Stringaris et al., 2009c). This impairment was not just due to the presence of other disorders, but seemed to be specific to mood lability. In the 20-year follow-up study (Stringaris et al., 2009a), adolescents who had shown irritability were less likely to have a higher degree, were more likely to be unemployed, and earned less money at outcome. This impairment in social role was independent of the presence of other disorders.

Chapter 6

Neuroscience of irritability

This chapter describes the brain structures and functions that are thought to be involved in the expression and regulation of angry emotions. It puts the associated brain activity in the context of processing emotions generally. Fig. 6.1 indicates some of the structures in the brain that take part in the expression and regulation of anger, with particular reference to serotoninergic systems.

In broad terms, angry emotions are served by networks involving the appraisal of threatening and frustrating situations (e.g. the frontal cortex), the attaching of emotional valence (e.g. the amygdala, nucleus accumbens, limbic system), the dissemination of responsiveness and arousal (e.g. via monoamines and other chemicals released from nerve cells situated in the upper part of the brainstem), and the generation of rage reactions (e.g. from the hypothalamus).

This chapter will focus on the following questions:

- Is there a neural signature of irritability?
- How do children's brains process emotions?
- Do children with irritability have different neural and neurochemical responses from typically developing children?

Neurological processes

Affective aggression in humans and animals

The term 'irritability' is rarely used in the animal literature. Defensive or reactive aggression, however, is conceptually close to irritability (see Chapter 4) and can be helpful in understanding the brain networks involved.

In the cat, as in other animals, aggression can be induced by electrical stimulation of areas in the hypothalamus, as can be seen in Fig. 6.2. Within the area from the ventromedial hypothalamic nucleus through to the lateral hypothalamus there are two distinct areas which when stimulated may lead to two distinct types of aggression (Siegel et al., 1999). Stimulation of the medial portion of the hypothalamus—close to the ventromedial nucleus—causes defensive or affective aggression. This form of aggression,

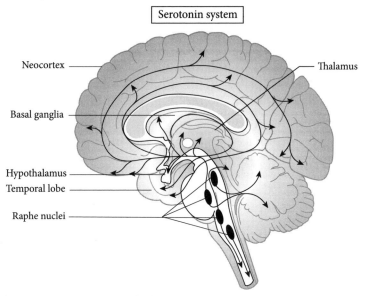

Fig. 6.1 Serotonin systems in the brain.

known for many years as 'affektive Abwehrreaktion' is characterized in the cat by pilorection (hair-raising), dilatation of the pupils, arching of the back, and unsheathing of the claws. Similar emotional responses can be elicited in rats (Haller, 2013) and mice (Dayu et al., 2011), but there are differences in the precise anatomical sites of the response and its elicitation.

This form of aggression with its marked arousal stands in marked contrast to the quiet biting attack which is produced by stimulation of more lateral hypothalamic sites (see Fig. 6.2). It is characteristic of a proactive form of aggression, such as when a cat launches a quiet attack on its victim, for example a rat (Wasman et al., 1962; Siegel et al., 1999). This instrumental attack may have more in common with human proactive aggression.

In humans, natural experiments suggest some similarities with other animals. In the past psychosurgery was used in some countries to treat severe forms of aggression. Case series of such surgical interventions supported a role for the hypothalamus in anger and aggression. Sano et al. (1970), for instance, reported that stimulation of the posterior hypothalamus in 51 patients with pathologically aggressive behaviour caused increases in blood pressure and heart rate and dilation of the pupils. Surgical lesions through electrocauterization of hypothalamic areas exerted calming effects on the individuals. Furthermore, tumours of the hypothalamus can cause rage-like behaviours as well as laughing spells (Savard et al., 2003).

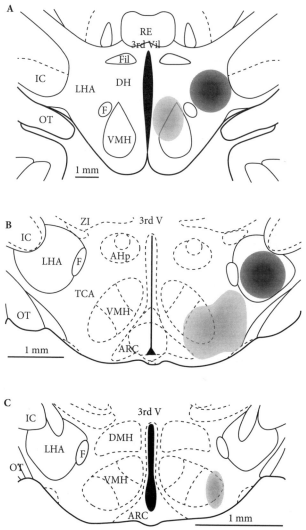

Fig. 6.2 Aggression-related hypothalamic areas in the cat (A), rat (B), and mouse (C). Defensive rage (light grey) and quiet biting (dark grey) areas arising from electrical stimulation experiments in the cat and their equivalents in the rat and mouse are depicted.

Reprinted from Brain Res Bull, 93, Haller, J, The neurobiology of abnormal manifestations of aggression—a review of hypothalamic mechanisms in cats, rodents, and humans, 97–109, Copyright 2013, with permission from Elsevier.

More generally, a threat network encompassing the amygdala, hypothalamus, and the periaqueductal grey is thought to underlie affective aggression (Blair, 2013). In humans, the threat network appears to be stimulated by fear-provoking stimuli, such as the presentation of a tarantula spider (Mobbs et al., 2010). Indeed, evidence suggests that components of the threat network, particularly the amygdala, are active in young people with conduct problems prone to non-proactive aggression (Jones et al., 2009). Current theory (Rolls, 2007) based on animal experiments suggests that whether presentation of a threat will result in an individual escaping (flight) or fighting will depend on the intensity of the stimulus and the environmental contingencies available to them. If there is a way to escape, flight will occur. If, however, there is no escape in sight, the threatened individual will be more likely to engage in reactive aggression.

These fascinating findings suggest that the hypothalamus, periaqueductal grey, and amygdala are sites of generation of aggression in animals and possibly in humans. Yet, there are still open questions. First, the role of the hypothalamus in aggression has not been conclusively demonstrated in functional studies of the living human—the calming of the aggressive individuals following surgery could have been due to the experience of being subjected to psychosurgery. Improvements in the resolution of neuroimaging may address this problem. Secondly, we know little about the feelings that accompany aggression in humans (and animals for that matter). Hypothalamic rage used to be described as sham rage or as pseudoaffective. Thirdly, it is unclear whether stimulation of the areas that lead to affective aggression in animals might be areas which could also give rise to flight responses. In fight and flight animals show the sort of arousal that arises from hypothalamic stimulation as already described. Can the neural processes of anger, rage, and irritability be distinguished from each other and from fear? Experiments with humans that vary environmental contingencies in such a way as to distinguish between aggression and fear have yet to be conducted. Moreover, the theory will need to account for some inter-individual differences. There are children who are very anxious and fear-prone yet hardly ever manifest aggression, and anxious children who are very likely to be aggressive. The origins of these inter-individual differences may well be related to temperament as well as social learning, and may be underlain by frontal cortical regulatory functions.

Anger, irritability, and basic emotions

More than a century of psychological research has shown that emotions can be defined in various and often overlapping ways, and that each of these definitions has its merits and limitations (Kagan, 2004; Stringaris, in press). This is clearest in the debate surrounding basic emotions. Our language recognizes a number of different emotions such as anger sadness, and joy. Some authorities claim the existence of a basic set of emotions (Ekman et al., 2011). The basic emotion view has certain affinities (Barrett, 2011) with Darwin's project on identifying universal and innate expressions in humans and animals. Basic emotions are said to be characterized by distinctive universal signals (e.g. facial expressions) and distinctive physiology, distinctive subjective experience, and the fact that they are present in humans as well as other primates (Ekman et al., 2011). Typical examples according to these authors are anger, disgust, fear, joy, surprise, and success.

However, this basic emotions view has been challenged on conceptual (Ortony et al., 1990), physiological (Frankenhaeuser, 1971), and anthropological (Jack et al., 2012) grounds. Indeed it seems that only subjective accounts and behaviour (such as approach or withdrawal) may distinguish between sadness and anger. These two emotions cannot be distinguished on the basis of either physiology or cognitive biases (Lench et al., 2011; Lindquist et al., 2013) Moreover, in a recent meta-analysis of brain regions involved in emotion processing it proved difficult to identify any neural substrate specific to a given emotion (Lindquist et al., 2012). One of the few exceptions has been the linking of the left orbitofrontal cortex (OFC) with anger. However, in that meta-analysis, brain correlates of anger were not restricted to the OFC but extended to other areas of the frontal lobe.

Some have suggested that it makes little sense to search for the brain correlates of anger (Lindquist et al., 2012) and that our common words to describe emotions may not map exactly onto brain function (LeDoux, 2000). However, human beings do distinguish between emotions and do feel irritable and recognize others' anger. Such phenomena must have a physiological basis, so the question remains about how brain responses of anger are shaped.

Environment, contingencies, and rewards

It is very likely that our understanding of physiology is simply not advanced enough to discover what distinguishes irritability from other emotions such as fear. Also, distinguishing between them may require taking the environment into account. General arousal may be shared between negative emotions: pilorection, pupillary dilation, and tachycardia may be common to anger and fear. Their differentiation may depend on the environmental contingencies that shape the response, and the associated conditions of reward and punishment.

Perhaps searching for brain areas that specialize in specific categories of emotions or behaviours is futile—brain function is more economical than a one-to-one relationship between each emotional state and a brain region would require (Rolls, 2007). Instead, the brain may have evolved to respond flexibly to variations in the environment. Emotions are part of that ability to respond—especially to respond rapidly, before full and detailed intellectual appraisal or in its absence. Immediate brain responses to frustration would need to include: shifting to new processes, reallocating attention, and generating and controlling heightened responsiveness.

Research is advancing fast and it is too soon for definitive conclusions. There are nevertheless some useful formulations that are relevant to clinicians. Rolls (2007) proposes that emotions are states that are elicited by rewards or punishers, which he calls instrumental reinforcers. Rewards are appetitive stimuli (those that bring about pleasure), while punishers are aversive stimuli bringing about unpleasant states. According to Rolls' theory, different emotions will be elicited according to which reinforcer is present.

The theory can be usefully extended to include the intensity of the reinforcer (the value of the reward), the presence of multiple—even opposing—reinforcers, the presence of secondary reinforcers (such as pre-existing cognitive appraisals), and crucially the behavioural responses available to the individual (is resistance futile, or could anger bring about a reward?) (Rolls, 2007). In this sense anger would arise under the combination of two things: the *omission of an expected reward* at a time when an *active behavioural response* is possible (Rolls, 2007).

This is accomplished by the convergence of sensory information (e.g. smell, touch, taste) into a brain area computing the reward value of such reinforcers, typically the OFC. Then other areas of the OFC and the amygdala mediate the learning of associations between neutral primary re-stimuli (e.g. a smell) and primary reinforcers. Such information would generate patterns of autonomic (e.g. tachycardia via the hypothalamus) or motor (e.g. fight, via the striatum) responses. The ability of the OFC to calculate the reward value of stimuli—and by extension influence behavioural, autonomic, and cognitive outcomes—has prompted people to describe it as a regulator of emotions. Perhaps inter-individual variation in how this regulator operates could explain why some people are angrier than others.

Anger regulation

What makes some people angrier than others? So far we have learnt that anger may be generated in those evolutionarily ancient parts of the brain like the periaqueductal grey matter (Mobbs et al., 2007), the amygdala, and the hypothalamus. We have also seen that the phylogenetically more recent OFC may calculate the value of stimuli and thus shape autonomic and behavioural responses. Chapter 4 has distinguished between the intensity of anger and the processes that regulate it. Does excessive activity of the subcortical areas such as the hypothalamus make people prone to irritability; or is it some deficit in regulation by the OFC and related areas?

Answers to these questions are not yet definitive. Research has mostly focused on neuroimaging techniques such as functional magnetic resonance imaging (fMRI). In fMRI the activation of brain regions is measured by analysing the effects of a strong magnetic field on radio waves passing through the brain. The interference that results is modified by naturally occurring magnets in the brain, such as the iron–oxygen bond in haemoglobin, and therefore by the arrival of oxygenated blood to an active area. This has been the technique used in children because of its safety—there is no exposure to ionizing radiation involved.

Unfortunately, however, using techniques such as fMRI to measure activity in the hypothalamus is more difficult than measuring activity in the neocortex. Activation in the amygdala is easier to measure, but its relationship to anger is complex. The amygdala is activated by threat cues (such as threatening faces), but people prone to anger may actually show diminished responses to negatively valenced emotional stimuli (Brotman et al., 2010). By contrast, there is clearer evidence that deficient regulation in the OFC may result in anger. Recently, Blair (2012) has proposed that anger may be the result of deficient regulation by the OFC. Indeed, patients with lesions in this area are at higher risk for impulsive, socially inappropriate behavior and irritability (Rolls et al., 1994).

These patients with frontal damage were much more likely than other patients to make perseverative errors in a response reversal task. In response reversal tasks, stimuli that were once rewarded with money, for example for touching the correct pattern on a computer screen, stop becoming rewarding (the subject may actually lose money). Patients with damage to the OFC continued to make responses to stimuli that were no longer rewarding and reported that they felt unable to inhibit this response. Interestingly, children with chronic irritability also seem to have deficits in tasks that require cognitive flexibility, that is an ability to adapt thoughts and actions changes in environmental contingencies (Dickstein et al., 2007).

Neural processing in children with chronic irritability

The type of psychopathology to which irritability is most central is DMDD. This disorder, recently defined in DSM-5, applies only to children and young people up to the age of 18 years and consists of severe irritability in combination with dysphoria between outbursts. That chronic dysphoria is compounded of anger and distress (see Chapter 12). The diagnostic definition is based on the previous idea of SMD. Most of the imaging research on irritability has been done in young people with SMD. It has implicated processes subserving cognitive flexibility, and responses to reward and punishment.

Cognitive flexibility and reward

Dickstein and colleagues from Ellen Leibenluft's laboratory at the National Institute of Mental Health in the United States have shown that children with SMD perform worse than typically developing controls in tasks that tap response reversal (Dickstein et al., 2007). (This deficit did not seem specific to the diagnosis: young people with bipolar disorder—who may also be irritable—also found it more difficult to stop responding to stimuli that were not being rewarded.)

Adleman and colleagues from the same lab used a response reversal task in an fMRI scanner to examine whether the low performance of young people with bipolar disorder and SMD compared with controls was due to the same or different neural processes (Adleman et al., 2011). They found that both SMD and bipolar groups differed significantly from healthy volunteers. Healthy youth showed increased activity in the striatum when they made errors—this increase in activity is normative, probably dependent on dopamine, and reflects the important ability to learn from such errors (Packard et al., 2002). However, in addition to this, children with SMD also failed to show an increase in neural activity in the inferior frontal gyrus (IFG) (part of which overlaps with the OFC) which children with bipolar disorder and healthy volunteers showed. Neural activity in the IFG during response conflict—as when subjects made errors in this task—probably reflects control over motor responding (Budhani et al., 2007). Indeed, activity in the IFG increases according to the control demands of a situation (Dodds et al., 2011). The authors speculated that their findings may indicate a chronic frontostriatal dysfunction in those with SMD; by contrast people with bipolar disorder, when they are euthymic (as they were in this particular study), seem to benefit from an intact IFG.

Frustration

The response reversal task probes cognitive flexibility; however, it is not designed to elicit emotional states that are characteristic of irritability. Frustration tasks, as the name implies, are designed to do precisely that. In the Affective Posner task, probands take part in a game that is rigged to make them feel that they perform badly—they end up not getting rewards that they were made to expect during the game. Such tasks have a number of effects. First, they cause frustration and therefore arousal—given what we have said previously, the expectation is that subcortical areas, particularly the amygdala, would become activated. Secondly, these tasks place a demand on attentional resources. As we have noted with regard to children's development in Chapter 4, shifting one's attention away from frustrating events is an important part of emotion regulation. This involves prefrontal regions, such as the IFG, and the parietal cortex. Thirdly, because this task involves the processing of reward and punishment (remember, failing to get a reward is called a punishment here), one would expect activations in the OFC. The ventral striatum should also be involved—it is considered to be for the limbic structures what the neostriatum is for neocortical structures, namely a route for limbic structures to reach output regions. The ventral striatum receives input from the amygdala and the OFC and projects to the ventral pallidum and this influences regions such as the subthalamic nucleus.

Deveney and her colleagues from Leibenluft's laboratory used the Affective Posner task to compare young people with SMD with age-matched healthy volunteer youngsters while their brains were being imaged in the scanner (Deveney et al., 2013). As expected, children with SMD reported more frustration than healthy controls during the frustration part of the task. Frustration seems to disrupt attention—both groups were about 30% less accurate than during the non-frustrating parts of the task. Both groups of children were also slower to respond during invalid trials (that is trials where the cue and target were in opposite locations) than during valid trials; however, children with SMD were also significantly slower than healthy volunteers to respond to invalid trials. This suggests that children with SMD may have particular difficulties with shifting attention when they are frustrated.

The neural basis of these behavioural results may be reflected in what Deveney et al. (2013) found during the fMRI task. Areas in the posterior parietal lobe of children with SMD were less active during negative feedback trials of the frustration task than in healthy volunteers. The parietal lobe is involved in selective attention, that is, the preferential processing of a subset of information (Behrmann et al., 2004). Interestingly, underactivation in this area that is involved in higher cognitive processing was accompanied by underactivation in the amygdala and the striatum during negative feedback trials.

So far, the results suggest that children with SMD find it difficult to adapt to changes in environmental contingencies. The findings of the response reversal task suggest that cognitive rigidity may be an underlying trait in children with SMD, while in the Affective Posner task those children are more easily frustrated and have more attention lapses. The neuropsychological findings of these studies are in keeping with the predictions of Rolls' theory of emotion and the predictions of Blair about anger generation. However, the brain findings are only partly in line with predictions. As expected, children with SMD failed to show the normative increases in activity in the striatum and the OFC during failed trials in the response reversal task. However, no frontal abnormalities were detected in the Affective Posner task, although this may be due to a lack of power.

Perhaps the most puzzling finding from the Affective Posner task is the hypoactivity of the amygdala. According to standard theory, the amygdala is a structure typically activated by arousal, frustration, or stress. Indeed, this is a well-replicated finding throughout studies employing stress- or frustration-related paradigms. It therefore may seem odd that there should be hypo- rather than hyperactivation of the amygdala, raising the question whether the finding has occurred by chance or is due to task-specific confounds.

However, Brotman et al. (2010) observed similar hypoactivation of the amygdala in young people with SMD who were asked to rate their fear of neutral faces. Compared with healthy volunteers (and with children with bipolar disorder) the left amygdala of children with severe irritability was less active, whereas children with ADHD showed hyper-responsive left amygdala. Similar hypoactivation of the amygdala has been found in children with depression (Beesdo et al., 2009) when viewing emotional faces. This is particularly interesting given the longitudinal and genetic links that exist between irritability and depression (see Chapter 5). Could amygdala hypoactivation represent one of the underlying mechanisms that link irritable and depressed moods? This is a difficult question to answer, not least because of an inherent limitation in fMRI research—the lack of an absolute baseline. This means that in this case the relative hyporeactivity of the amygdala could also have been caused because children with SMD showed increased activation in the part of the task that has been used as a baseline, namely the question about 'how wide is the nose?'.

Summary of neural processing in children with irritability

This survey of the functional imaging literature of children with irritability points to three probably interconnected neural characteristics. First, the difficulties in dealing with changing environmental contingencies may be reflected in the failure of children with SMD to activate the IFG during a response reversal task. Secondly, it emerges that responding to changing environmental contingencies may be more difficult for children with SMD because their ability to reallocate attentional resources diminishes as they become frustrated. This inability may be reflected in the hypoactivation of the parietal lobe observed during the frustration task. Thirdly, children with SMD seem to have an unexpected amygdalal response to frustration but also to the emotional judgement of faces. This last finding raises an important question about how mood may dampen typical emotional responses. It leads to a more general question about distinctions between mood and emotion.

Mood changes

In Chapter 2 we discussed the importance of considering time-scales when thinking about mood, and irritability in particular. Most of this book deals with what is termed chronic irritability, and the neural signatures previously discussed concern those children with chronic irritability. However, while clinical research has been mindful of those time-scales, neuroscience research rarely considers them. The two most obvious questions are: first, what determines chronicity (we can all get irritable, but what makes some people be irritable for much longer) and, secondly, what are the effects of chronicity? The answers to these questions are relevant to how a person will respond to environmental contingencies and, indeed, which environments this person may select or evoke. The same questions can be asked of other mood disorders, such as depression or mania. The determinants of chronicity remain unclear for most mood disorders, while the situation remains unclear about the effects of chronicity in depression and mania. It is encouraging that duration effects are beginning to be considered in the distinction between fear and anxiety. In this field researchers speak of the former as a response to phasic stress whereas anxiety is a response to sustained threat. Interestingly, the two can be distinguished on the basis of their neural pathways (Davis et al., 2010).

However, there are obvious methodological problems with studying chronicity. Functional imaging and electroencephalography measure brain changes on the time-scale of milliseconds to seconds. Most experimental paradigms are focusing on rapid changes in emotion perception (e.g. emotion processing), that is short-lived states, rather than persistent states or the formation of traits. For ethical reasons even experiments with mood induction last for only a short period of time. Therefore, the neural correlates of mood remain unclear (Rolls, 2007).

Neurotransmitter and neuromodulator effects on anger

The brain's responses to environmental changes are influenced strongly by chemicals with widespread influences on brain systems. Dopamine, serotonin (5-hydroxytryptamine), and noradrenaline (norepinephrine) all alter mood (Ruhe et al., 2007). These are all amines ('monoamines'), produced in cells in the upper part of the brainstem that project over large parts of the brain (serotonin cells from the raphe nuclei; see Fig. 6.1). When they are released from nerve terminals (synapses) they bind to several different specialized receptors on the surface of other nerve cells. The result is not usually to directly cause the receiving (post-synaptic) nerve cell to fire off an impulse, but to alter its disposition to react to other incoming signals.

The levels of dopamine, serotonin, and noradrenaline can therefore have a powerful effect on many functions of the brain, and they have been widely studied in many species of animals. Their production is sensitive to environmental changes, for instance via the actions of the amygdala and limbic system in processing emotionally charged stimuli and sending input to those cells in the upper brainstem that are projecting widely and determining neurotransmitter release (Phillips et al., 2003; Surguladze et al., 2003; Talarovicova et al., 2007). The levels and release of monoamines therefore provide a sensitive system through which messages about the changing environment can be conveyed to produce enduring but modifiable changes in motivated behaviour.

Low levels of *serotonin* can occur naturally, and can be produced experimentally—even in humans—by dietary changes that deplete it in the brain. They can be increased—again, in humans—by antidepressant drugs such as fluoxetine. Experiments indicate that low levels are associated with persisting states of anger, as well as with other negative mood states such as depression (Seo et al., 2008), and that increasing levels are associated with reductions in impulsive aggression (Silva et al., 2007). A variant of a gene influencing serotonin, the serotonin transporter promoter *5HTTLPR*, has been linked to high levels of hostility as assessed by a personality questionnaire (Keltikangas-Jarvinen et al., 2009). The mechanisms by which lowered serotonin induces irritability remain unclear, and the strengths of the findings are variable and depend on the methods by which serotonin is probed (Duke et al., 2013). Moreover, in animal models of aggression—such as the social dominance model of rats—drugs acting on serotoninergic systems alter aggression in unexpected ways. Some findings suggest that higher, rather than lower, levels of brain serotonin may contribute to aggression (de Boer et al., 2005; Biederman, 2006).

Dopamine has been implicated strongly in the processes involved in cognitive flexibility, attention, and reward—all of which have been considered as factors in the elicitation of anger. Dopamine levels are also considered to contribute to several psychiatric disorders, including schizophrenia and ADHD. The influences on aggression are complex, and those on irritability specifically are obscure. Drugs that increase dopamine levels in the striatum reduce both overt and covert aggression in young people with ADHD (Connor et al., 2002). Drugs that antagonize its action are widely used in the treatment of aggressive and hostile behaviours (see Chapter 14). (In a study in mice by Couppis and Kennedy (2008), a dopamine antagonist reduced the rewarding effect of aggression; and possibly this could be a mechanism of therapeutic change.)

Noradrenaline levels are considered to be linked to levels of arousal and anxiety.

Several attempts have been made to link individual monoamines with specific dimensions of emotion (e.g. Lövheim (2012), in whose formulation a disposition to rage would represent low serotonin, high dopamine, and high noradrenaline) or with responses to novelty, aversive stimuli, and reward (Cloninger et al., 1993). These attempts do of course recognize the oversimplifications involved. For one thing, manipulations of monoamine levels tend to have other and mixed effects on other systems. For another, the systems interact with each other and are subject to feedback. Importantly, the effects of monoamines do not depend only on the amount available to or released at the synapse. There are many types of receptors and the effects depend upon the type of receptor that is available to be stimulated.

Clinical aspects

The complexity of systems underlying anger and irritability means that they can be disrupted in many different ways. *Diffuse* brain lesions very often cause people to become irritable. Acquired brain injuries, dementias, and encephalopathies can all upset the control of anger. It is, however, usually profitless to investigate for a *localized* lesion even when problems appear for the first time on a background of typical development. The exceptions are mentioned in Chapter 13.

Neuroscience is uncovering some mechanisms involved, and in time this may well give us some clues on how to intervene. The most immediate seems likely to be the development of new drugs, or better use of existing ones. Clinicians, however, are sometimes tempted to prescribe drugs based on a speculative understanding of the brain regions and monoamines that they believe to be involved. This can lead them into experimental treatments that lack an evidence base and can be harmful. The neuroscience described in this chapter is advancing rapidly, but is not yet at the stage where it should govern decisions about the treatment of individual patients. Rather, treatments based on neurobiological understanding should follow the evidence base—and especially the results of clinical trials, as described in the following chapters.

Chapter 7

ADHD and irritability

ADHD is a common problem. Polanczyk et al. (2007) suggested a prevalence in schoolchildren of about 5%, but with very wide disparities between countries in the rate with which it is recognized. In the current edition of the American Psychiatric Association's *Diagnostic and Statistical Manual of Mental Disorders* (DSM-5) the core features are inattention, overactivity, and impulsiveness. In the World Health Organization's scheme (ICD-10) there are the same core features, but the name applied is 'hyperkinetic disorder', the criteria are more strictly applied, and the prevalence is only about one-quarter of that of ADHD. *Inattention* describes lack of concentration on detail, a short attention span in unmotivating situations, forgetfulness, distractibility in situations requiring focus on a task, and a slapdash attitude. *Overactivity* describes an excess of movement in situations requiring calm. *Impulsiveness* refers to poorly controlled activity—resulting in accident-proneness, impatience, intrusiveness, and hasty, inept decision-making. ADHD is very often accompanied by oppositional–defiant behaviour problems, but they are separate forms of disturbance, as illustrated in Box 7.1 (see also Chapter 9).

Strength and nature of the association

Children with ADHD are often emotionally labile. Many of them react unpredictably and with great intensity, but transiently, to events affecting them. The emotion is appropriate, but its expression is excessive. Irritability is a characteristic part of this lability, with tantrums that are extreme and easily provoked, but lasting at most for a few hours.

For some time the association between irritability and syndromes of hyperactivity was simply a matter of definition. During the era of 'minimal brain function' in the 1930s and of 'hyperactive child syndrome' in the years between 1950 and 1980, lability of mood was a key part of descriptions of the disorder. The situation changed in 1980 with the appearance of the third revision of the American Psychiatric Association's *Diagnostic and Statistical Manual of Mental Disorders* (DSM-III). The criteria for 'attention deficit disorder with hyperactivity' (ADDH) were then formulated to comprise

---

Box 7.1 A child with both ADHD and conduct problems

Jack is a 9-year-old boy with a diagnosis of ADHD and specific learning difficulties. His mother says that 'he can be a nightmare', he 'paces around all the time, can't sit still', and he 'gets into fights all the time' with his brother. He shouts back at his mother and his aunt when they try to stop him from running around: 'I bargain with him, I shout at him, nothing works really'. He is known to be grumpy, especially on school days—he gets picked on by other pupils and he gets into fights which leads to him being excluded from school. Even a slight remark by his brother is enough to make him very angry. He describes himself as 'naughty' and tells you that 'sometimes my anger is too much'. Jack's ADHD symptoms improved considerably on methylphenidate, but his anger somewhat less so. He also benefitted from subsequent school interventions to stop the bullying and his mother found that a reward chart was helpful.

---

inattention, impulsivity, and hyperactivity, in line with the beginnings of neuropsychological formulations of the disorder. Nevertheless, 'increased mood lability, low frustration tolerance, and temper outbursts' were all listed as associated features of ADDH. Diagnostic studies tended not to focus on the overlap. Irritability was usually studied only as an inherent part of the syndrome.

When research turned to the analysis of component behaviours rather than diagnostic syndromes, it appeared that irritability was not a part of the core cluster of symptoms that could be regarded as features of ADHD. Many applications of factor analysis to parent and teacher rating scales were carried out; meta-analysis distinguished robustly between components of impulsivity/overactivity and inattention on the one hand and disruptive behaviour on the other (NICE, 2008). Irritability was part of the latter. More specifically, epidemiological studies using rating scales that included 'irritability' as an item found that it associated with items such as fighting and disobedience rather than inattention and restlessness—for instance, in analyses of Rutter's teacher and parent rating scales in a sample of more than 3000 7-year-old boys in England (Taylor et al., 1991). Similarly, exploratory factor analysis of Conners' rating scales by Taylor and Sandberg (Taylor et al., 1984) in the UK, and by Ho et al. (1996) of the Rutter scales in a Hong Kong Chinese population found that temper outbursts and rapidly changing moods came out in a factor including defiance and uncooperativeness rather than one with inattentiveness and restlessness.

Irritable mood therefore became something of a diagnostic orphan. Temper tantrums themselves were included as one of the specific criteria for the diagnosis of 'oppositional disorder' which is separate from, but also frequently associated with, ADHD.

Irritability therefore needs to be seen as somewhat different from the core ADHD features. It can be thought of in dimensional terms as one of several *components* that contribute to psychopathology, along with dimensions such as inattentiveness and anxiety. As such it is often included as a part of 'emotional dysregulation' or 'emotional lability' (see Chapter 2).

Shaw et al. (2014) provide a review of epidemiological and clinical studies of the association between ADHD and emotional lability. Thirty-eight per cent of children with ADHD in a population survey showed marked emotional lability (Stringaris et al., 2009c)—a rate ten times that of the population as a whole. Furthermore, this form of emotional dysregulation predicted a more adverse outcome for ADHD in the same study.

Rates are comparably high in referred cases at clinics. Ambrosini et al. (2013) assessed 500 clinically referred ADHD subjects (mean age about 10 years) with the childhood version of the Schedule for Affective Disorder and Schizophrenia (K-SADS) and found that irritability characterized 21% of them. Sobanski et al. (2010), in a clinically referred population of 216 children with ADHD, applied a strict definition of emotional lability, namely three standard deviations or more above population norms on a scale from the Conners ratings. On this basis, 25% were emotionally labile as well.

In both the studies, the symptoms of emotional lability constituted an important additional clinical problem, and were strongly associated with additional diagnoses, especially depression and a pattern of dysthymic and oppositional problems. Furthermore, symptoms of emotional lability seem to be associated with poorer social outcome and peer rejection in children with ADHD (Maedgen et al., 2000). Conversely, the vast majority of cases with the severe condition of DMDD (see Chapter 12) occur in children who also show ADHD (Reddy et al., 2000).

It seems that the presence of poorly controlled emotion—including irritability—is both a strong association and a piece of extra and important clinical information about likely prognosis and possible causality. Furthermore, the specific symptom of irritability is very common in ADHD. Geller et al. (2002), using detailed research interview techniques, found very high rates of irritability: irritability was present in some 72% of children with ADHD. No doubt differences in referral patterns will make a difference to the profiles of cases seen.

Why are so many children with ADHD irritable?

The link between irritability and ADHD is not due only to the many arte-facts that can produce misleading correlations in series of referred cases. It is found in epidemiological studies of representative samples. Some of it can come from misdiagnosis. It is possible for a child's temper outbursts to be described in a way that leads to their being categorized in terms, such as 'impulsive', that lead the unwary to a diagnosis of ADHD even though the core features of ADHD are not present. This diagnostic trap can be avoided by en-suring that a clear history is taken of the child's behaviour and concentration between episodes of anger.

Developmental mechanisms

Several developmental processes can lead to a child with ADHD developing frequent tempers. They are not mutually exclusive and several pathways may be involved.

Evocative transactions

First, ADHD may create the provocations to others that lead them to re-spond with hostility and criticism and thus evoke anger in the child (Rutter et al., 1997). This represents a transactional chain which can be influenced by qualities of both the child and the parents (and siblings, teachers, and peers). It is unlikely to be due only to a gene–environment correlation, because a study of monozygotic twins (whose genes are, of course, the same) has found that their exposure to hostile expressed emotion predicts the extent to which they become hostile themselves (Caspi et al., 2004).

An idea of whether this is happening in an individual case can be obtained by enquiring about the details of what happens in disciplinary interactions. Sometimes it is possible to observe it in family situations. It is also possible to assess hostility and criticism from the emotional tone of an interview. Hos-tility and criticism may be a target for therapeutic intervention in their own right—possibly through psychoeducation (Ferrin et al., 2011) and possibly through medication of the child, which does indeed reduce hostile parent-expressed emotion (Schachar et al., 1987).

Dyscontrol

Secondly, the dyscontrol of activity and attention that is characteristic of ADHD (Taylor et al., 2008) might be closely related to a deficient control of emotions including anger. ADHD is associated with altered functioning of at least some of the neurocognitive processes considered in Chapter 6 as contributions to poor control of anger and other emotions. Decreased ventral striatal activity during reward processing has been reported several times in ADHD by comparison with typically developing controls (Scheres et al., 2007; Strohle et al., 2008) and decreased prefrontal activation to the presentation of angry faces is described in ADHD (as well as in bipolar disorder) (Passarotti et al., 2010). It is therefore possible to conceive of both emotional volatility and the core ADHD symptoms as being a part of the same lack of inhibitory control. Such poor control might be responsible for the quick igniting of anger after frustration, with a rapid 'flash' of angry passion and an immediate translation of it into aggressive action. The poor control might also be a matter of failing to recover a state of equanimity after an episode of anger. In favour of this idea is a positive effect of stimulants on both cognitive and emotional dysregulation (Shaw et al., 2014)—but it could be that stimulants act on the two targets in very different ways. Against the idea—at least as a sole explanation—is the lack of any obvious difference between mood dysregulation in those with ADHD and those without, but this issue deserves systematic research.

Underlying risks in common

Thirdly, the association of ADHD and irritability may reflect their both being aspects of one set of underlying risks. Both, for instance, can certainly occur as features of brain damage or disorder; and both can probably be reflections of genetic factors. The family pattern of transmission was investigated by Surman et al. (2011), giving information about the association between ADHD and 'deficient emotional self-regulation' (DESR). They studied the siblings of adults with a diagnosis of ADHD. Those siblings had elevated rates of having ADHD, whether or not the proband had DESR as well. But they only had an elevated risk of DESR if the proband had DESR as well as ADHD. ADHD and DESR co-segregated. Within the siblings of people with both ADHD and DESR, those who had developed ADHD were the only ones who had also developed DESR.

This does not necessarily mean that the link is genetic—it might also be due to psychosocial processes in the family—such as the vicious cycle of aversive and hostile behaviours suggested. A genetic reason, however, is supported by a twin analysis reported by Merwood et al. (2014). They used measures intended to capture the similar concept of emotional lability and of core ADHD symptoms in a large sample of twins aged 5 to 18 years from the general population. When the similarities were compared between the monozygotic and dizygotic twins there was strong evidence for a single, genetically heritable factor accounting for the association. This is strong evidence for an intimate connection between the genetic risks for ADHD and for the low-level problems of emotional dysregulation that are found in a community sample. It remains possible, in principle, that there is a different story for the very intense and persistent levels of irritability that would be found in psychiatric conditions such as DMDD or bipolar disorder. And it is quite possible that additional characteristics mediate the development of ADHD into emotional dysregulation—such as a version of a gene that may influence the child's emotional reaction to hostile levels of maternal or family-expressed emotion (Taylor et al., 2008).

Comorbidity with other disorders

Fourthly, and notwithstanding the aforementioned evidence, it is also possible that ADHD and irritability are quite separate kinds of problem and their association comes about because both are features of another disorder. This might particularly be the case when the irritability is at the intense level associated with affective illness, such as bipolar disorder or major depression (described in Chapters 10 and 12). Geller et al. (1998) examined this in a study aiming to differentiate the features of bipolar disorder from ADHD by a clinical comparison of the two disorders. They found that the symptom of irritability characterized ADHD without bipolar disorder just as much as it did bipolar disorder. (This was in contrast to core bipolar symptoms, such as euphoria and grandiosity, which were much more frequent in bipolar disorder than in uncomplicated ADHD.)

Nevertheless, and in spite of the evidence favouring irritability and emotional dysregulation as inherent parts of, or complications of, ADHD, clinicians should be alert to the individual cases where the extreme intensity of irritability or its episodicity make an additional diagnosis of bipolar disorder or DMDD tenable. There may be different types of irritability, with different implications for comorbidity in ADHD. The way that the questions about irritability are phrased may make a considerable difference to the pattern of results. For example, Mick et al. (2005) asked 247 children with ADHD the questions which operationalized 'irritability' from the different modules of the K-SADS structured interview. From the depression module, the question is: 'Has there ever been a period of two weeks or longer in which you were feeling mad (or cranky) most of the day nearly every day?'. From the mania module, the question is: 'Have you ever had a period of one week or longer when you felt super angry, grouchy, or cranky (or irritable) all of the time?'. From the ODD module, the questions are: 'Do you often lose your temper?', 'Are you often angry or resentful?', and 'Is it easy to make you mad or to annoy you?'. When these different questions were tabulated against the diagnoses made with the same interview then they did tend to segregate with the appropriate diagnosis. For example the 'super angry' item was present in 23 out of 30 of the young people who received the comorbid diagnosis of 'bipolar disorder', but in only 11 out of 144 of those with ADHD who had no comorbid mood disorder diagnosis. The less strict questions from the ODD module were, by contrast, present in a majority of those with ADHD, even when no mood disorder was diagnosed.

A clinical implication, which is in keeping with recommendations made about the mood disorder DMDD in Chapter 12, is that very severe levels of irritability are grounds for a comorbid diagnosis, while minor levels can be seen as being part of, or having developed from, ADHD itself (usually in combination with oppositional disorder). These 'minor' levels can still be both very common and very disabling, but do not usually justify a separate diagnosis.

Management of irritability in people with ADHD

Detecting irritability in ADHD

The initial assessment (see Chapter 3) will establish whether irritability and dysregulated mood are in fact abnormal in intensity and duration, are out of keeping with the developmental age of the child, and are attributable to any stresses and frustrations under which the children might be living, including harsh physical punishment (Caspi et al., 2002). The next step is to assess the presence or absence of other mental health problems known to cause extreme irritability, notably autism and autism-related disorders, and abuse of psychoactive drugs.

Detecting ADHD in irritability

For this purpose, the key is the recognition of inattention and impulsiveness. Rating scales from parents and teachers are a useful screen, but interviews with parents and children, and observation of children, are needed to make sure that inattention and impulsiveness are present at times when the emotional symptoms are not marked, and that they are not due to rater biases such as halo effects or misunderstanding of words.

Assessing reciprocal influences of ADHD and irritability

A further step for those whose irritability and volatility of mood are indeed developmentally inappropriate, disproportionate to the provocations, and accompanied by core ADHD features could be to consider how far they are a direct result of the poor self-control that ADHD entails rather than the other developmental pathways mentioned. In practice, however, this is difficult and often misleading. Reconstructing the biography and course of problems is dependent on recall and subject to the reconstructions of memory.

The practical question is likely to be whether alleviation of the ADHD is also helpful for the irritability problem. Accordingly, an early step in therapy is to control the core features of ADHD, and then to reassess how much irritability remains and whether it needs attention in its own right.

Psychological interventions

The general psychological management of excessive anger is described in Chapter 14, and remains appropriate in the presence of ADHD. Some modifications may be necessary to take account of the particular problems of ADHD.

1 Psychoeducation about the nature of the condition is strongly valued by sufferers and their families (Ferrin et al., 2011). Simply the recognition of ADHD as a cause, as a medical condition rather than a moral failure, and as a potentially treatable condition, can help a family to forgive itself and liberate its problem-solving skills.

2 Withdrawal of reward is often ineffective as a therapeutic procedure. This is not only because of the initial worsening of problem behaviours (as set out in Chapter 14), but also because of the experimental findings in children with ADHD (and/or other kinds of disruptive behaviour) that extinction is slow and may be incomplete.

3 Speed and novelty of reward are of particular importance in drawing up behavioural programmes. Both children with ADHD and animal models such as the spontaneously hypertensive rat show a rapid decline in the effect of rewards on behaviour with increasing delay of reward (Sagvolden et al., 2005). This would encourage the use of procedures such as timers, set to go off after certain periods of anger-free activity (e.g. playing peaceably with a sibling for 5 minutes), or rapidly noting occasions when anger has been controlled, and coming in with a reward (or announcement of a reward) within a span of a few seconds. Similarly, the use of swiftly changing rewards would be sensible: for instance, one day applying the reward of playing with a parent, another day extra television time, another day a favourite food. Modifications such as these have not received formal trial, but are widely applied.

4 ADHD in a child is often accompanied by ADHD in a parent. Parents thus affected may have real problems in organizing for clinic attendance, and may need reminders and home visits. They may have particular problems in holding themselves back, and therefore find that advice to 'ignore minor tantrums' does not apply to their condition. Rather, they may find it easier to acquire skills in making positive responses rather than in withholding negative ones.

5 The attentional problems may make it harder for them to follow the cognitive approaches to anger control that are mentioned in Chapter 14. They may need the help of a teacher or family member to remember and engage in the homework practice that is involved.

Diet treatments

An extensive literature on the effect of removing artificial colourings and preservatives did not reach the scientific level required to establish it in the recommended treatment of ADHD (NICE, 2008). More recently, however, meta-analysis has established that there are indeed beneficial effects of excluding such substances from the diet (Sonuga-Barke et al., 2013). Furthermore, two randomized controlled trials in the general population of children have reported adverse behavioural effects of giving such substances (McCann et al., 2007). It is therefore worth revisiting the older studies and noting several reports that irritability improved even more characteristically than the core features of ADHD when the substances were withdrawn (Rowe and Rowe, 1994). Tartrazine has therefore been withdrawn by food manufacturers in the UK, and in the United States similar regulation is being considered by the Food and Drugs Administration. Effective labelling of foods and drinks makes it possible for families to avoid those containing additives.

Supplementation with minerals and vitamins does not yet have a solid evidence base, but the use of fish oil containing omega-3 polyunsaturated fatty acids does appear from meta-analysis of controlled trials to have a small but positive effect on many of the features of ADHD (Sonuga-Barke et al., 2013).

Drug treatments

The pharmacological treatment of irritability proceeds along rather different lines when ADHD is also present. The control of ADHD is usually the first step.

Stimulant medication and atomoxetine are the standard drug therapies for ADHD—and both can be expected to reduce emotional and aggressive symptoms as well as disruptive behaviours. Irritability has seldom been an explicit target for medication. Stimulant medication, however, can indeed modify the broader problem of emotional dysregulation. Shaw et al. (2014) identified six randomized controlled trials in children and five in adults that included measures reflecting emotional dysregulation. Methylphenidate had a modest but consistent positive action in comparison with placebo.

Using the data from a large controlled trial of medication against behavioural treatment of ADHD (MTA, 1999), Fernandez de la Cruz et al (Fernandez de la Cruz et al., 2014) recently found that medication treatment was superior to behavioural management but not to routine community care. Combining stimulants and behavioural treatment was better than community care or behavioural treatment alone, but not to medication alone. Moreover, the authors found that Irritability did not moderate the impact of treatment on parent- and teacher-reported ADHD symptoms in any of the 4 treatment groups. The authors concluded that treatments targeting ADHD symptoms were helpful for reducing irritability in children with ADHD and that irritability did not appear to worsen the response to treatment of ADHD.

Clinicians should also note the possibility that negative emotions may appear as a result of medication. Irritability is sometimes reported as an adverse effect of medication, but this may be a result of the condition rather than its treatment. Manos et al. (2011) reviewed the literature of reports from randomized trials, and found that while there were indeed some reports of irritability as an adverse effect, on balance stimulant medication was associated with a fall in irritability in comparison with placebo. The reduction was by 6.5% for parent ratings and 10.7% for teacher ratings, when the question was systematically asked (e.g. by an adverse events rating scale). A double-blind trial by Ahmann and colleagues (in Manos et al., 2011) focused on adverse events as the outcome; methylphenidate did indeed reduce irritability over the 7-day period of the trial.

Our clinical recommendation is that stimulant medication and atomoxetine in this comorbid situation are not contraindicated, and may well be helpful. The anti-ADHD drugs are relatively safe. Their adverse effects are usually minor and reversible by symptomatic treatment (Cortese et al., 2013). The contrast with the adverse effects of lithium, valproate, and the neuroleptics is striking enough to support the recommendation that the first line in drug management should be to control the ADHD, and then to review whether the irritability is sufficient to need further treatment.

Treatment with stimulants and atomoxetine should nevertheless be undertaken with enhanced monitoring and supervision in the comorbid situation. The frequency and intensity of anger should be recorded as a baseline measure, and again during regular monitoring.

Prescribing stimulants

The details of dose regimes do not differ from those recommended in uncomplicated ADHD. Methylphenidate is given in daily amounts of 5–60 mg. If an immediate-release formulation is chosen it should be given in divided doses through the day. Extended-release formulations, in beaded form, typically last up to 8 h; an osmotic-release preparation can last up to 12 h (and has a daily dosage range up to 72 mg). Prescription begins at the lower end of the range and builds up (e.g. by 10 mg a day each week) to the level giving the optimal combination of benefits and adverse effects. Some young people require, and can take safely, doses above the normal range. Where there is only a small response, and no adverse effects have appeared, then doses up to the equivalent of 100 mg of methylphenidate in a day have been regarded as reasonable by NICE (2008). Dexamfetamine doses are approximately half those of methylphenidate and last about as long. Lisdexamfetamine is longer-lasting—at least 12 h—and is given at a daily dose of 20–70 mg.

If the first drug given does not control the ADHD symptoms then recourse should be made to a second antihyperkinetic drug—atomoxetine or a different stimulant. Further treatment for ADHD beyond this level is not governed by a clear evidence base. Clonidine (0.05–0.4 mg daily) and guanfacine (1–4 mg daily) may be useful. They can both be mildly sedating, and this action may be of benefit in the very excitable and impulsive children who have been refractory in treatment so far. The choice of second-line drug may, however, be governed by the need to control high levels of anger and possibly aggression—and therefore to move to the mood stabilizing or antipsychotic drugs described in Chapter 14.

Further treatment

If the mood dysregulation persists despite control of the ADHD then behavioural approaches (anger control and parent training) should be considered, as in Cochrane Reviews for the treatment of aggressive and other conduct problems (Woolfenden et al., 2001). If these are not successful, or are inappropriate, and when the problems are sufficiently impairing to have an impact on the child's development, then further drug treatment should be considered (see Chapter 14). The question will be whether the adverse effects of the more potent drugs are outweighed by expectation of benefit.

Controlled trials do not yet give complete evidence on the balance of risk and benefit. Blader et al. (2009) conducted a randomized trial of divalproex (mean daily dose 567 mg) against placebo in 27 children and adolescents whose ADHD had been improved with stimulants but whose coexistent aggression was continuing to be a serious problem. The addition of divalproex to the stimulant regime was efficacious. Those treated with it met the criteria for remission of aggression more often than those who received placebo (in 8 out of 14 cases, compared with 2 out of 13 on placebo). The improvement was not attributable to further change in ADHD symptoms; the effect was more specifically on aggression. Aggression is not the same as irritability, but the combination of the two is frequent, distressing, and impairing.

Conversely, Scheffer et al. (2005) described how a stimulant could be a useful addition for controlling ADHD symptoms in 'paediatric bipolar disorder' after the chronic mood problem had been managed with divalproex.

Risperidone can also be effective for the broad problem of disruptive behaviour in children who are also being treated with stimulants for ADHD. Aman et al. (2004) reanalysed two randomized controlled trials (in children with subaverage IQ) and concluded that 'Risperidone was a safe and effective treatment, with or without a combined psychostimulant, for both disruptive behavior disorders and comorbid ADHD in children'.

Combination therapies have not often been evaluated rigorously, but they are called for in the severe, mixed, and complex cases where psychological management and monotherapy have been unsuccessful. Treatment advice for irritability and disruptive mood has to go beyond the scientific base, and should be read with corresponding caution. Caution should also be exercised by the prescriber, lest children are exposed to unreasonable risks from the medicines, and it should be explained to those responsible for the child that the medicines have not been rigorously assessed for efficacy or safety in ADHD.

If the irritability that coexists with ADHD is at the intensity, and with the episodicity, of a bipolar I disorder, then the advice to start with antihyperactivity treatment would be problematic (see Chapter 10). It is often said that stimulants can worsen mania. This does not necessarily apply (Scheffer et al., 2005), but vigilance is needed for deteriorating mood states and the possible need for co-prescription of a mood stabilizer.

Chapter 8

Irritability in autism spectrum disorders

Our understanding of autism has been changing, and the formulation of DSM-5 reflects this. Previously it was thought of as uncommon, severe, and characteristic—'nuclear autism' or 'Kannerian autism'—but with a penumbra of related conditions, termed variously 'pervasive developmental disorder', 'Asperger syndrome', 'pervasive refusal syndrome', and 'progressive disintegrative disorder'. The new DSM-5 revision, however, has drawn on research to consider that these are all parts of one 'autism spectrum'. It comprises two dimensions, one of deficits in social reciprocity and communication and one of restricted, repetitive behaviours (the latter often being termed a 'desire for sameness') (American Psychiatric Association, 2013). Both have to be present for the diagnosis. Other mental problems frequently coexist (see Box 8.1).

Size and nature of the association

Autism spectrum disorders (ASD) are present in about 11 children out of every thousand. They frequently coexist with emotional disorders, which were present in 44% of a population-based sample of 112 adolescents with ASD (Simonoff et al., 2008). Oppositional disorders, too, are frequent, and were found in about 28% of the epidemiologically ascertained series noted in Simonoff et al.

Anger is often a major problem presented to clinicians by people with ASD. Outbursts of rage are frequent events. Reports of series of children referred with ASD stress how common it is for irritability to be a problem, for example in 88% of the high-functioning and 84% of the low-functioning (i.e. with an IQ of less than 80) individuals in a report on 350 children with autism by Mayes et al (2011). Of course, it may well be that anger is a major reason for referral. Indeed, in the series of Mayes et al. irritability was also a problem in other conditions referred to that clinic—68% for those with intellectual retardation and 60% for those with brain injuries.

A non-referred series was described by Lecavalier (2006). He identified 487 children on the basis that the children were receiving educational

> ## Box 8.1 Anger in the spectrum of autism
>
> Johnny is a 12-year-old boy with a diagnosis of autism and mild learning difficulties. He has been attending his local child mental health clinic because of 'severe behaviour problems'. His mother describes that he can have 'outbursts' during which he 'he gets red in the face', 'tenses up', repeatedly screams 'I can't take it', and is in floods of tears. During such episodes he sometimes even smashes things or attacks his brother. During the most recent such outburst he destroyed his much-cherished Xbox. His tantrums can last for 3–4 hours. His mother is not sure about what triggers the outbursts. She notices that he is often grumpy for several hours before the tantrum and 'knackered' thereafter. His clinician conducts a functional analysis which reveals that these tantrums are usually related to imminent changes, such as family holidays, or visits by relatives.

services for 'pervasive developmental disorders' (i.e. the broad spectrum of autism): 19% were described as having a problem of irritability, 29% had tantrums, and 23% were 'explosive'.

Sometimes the frequency and severity of outbursts are so great that they need to be considered as a disorder in their own right—especially when they coexist with prolonged states of dysphoria. Severely unstable children were identified by Simonoff et al. (2012) in a series of 91 adolescents who had received a careful research diagnosis of ASD and who had been identified by screening a population of those with special educational needs and/or a clinical diagnosis. Their criteria for 'severe mood problems' were based on explosive rage, labile mood, low mood, and depressive thoughts, and were therefore similar (but not identical) to severe emotional dysregulation. Twenty-four of the 91 young people scored high on this measure. Those 24 also turned out to have high scores on questionnaire measures of emotional problems rated by both teachers and parents, but not on conduct problems or hyperactivity.

Why are so many children with autism spectrum disorders irritable?

There could, in theory, be several developmental routes through which children with ASD might come to be very irritable. Some of them have been tested by comparing the characteristics of autistic children with severe emotional dysregulation (Mikita et al, in press) or severe mood problems (Simonoff et al., 2012) with autistic children who do not show them.

The frustration that elicits anger may be very frequent, yet invisible to the rest of the family, if the provocation stems from interrupting the desire for sameness that is a key part of the condition. Lack of communicative ability may also be a powerful source of frustration. If there are difficulties in expressing one's needs clearly enough to be understood, then one suffers both from the unmet need and from the incomprehension of others. These are clearly going to be important triggers, but the extent to which people with autism vary in the intensity and frequency of anger is not necessarily determined by the level of these core autistic features of communication problems and the desire for sameness.

Irritability does not seem to be a core part of the condition itself. Simonoff et al. (2012) found that only parental ratings of severity of autism distinguished those with irritability from controls: clinician ratings did not, and neither did the diagnosis of whether they showed the full syndrome of 'nuclear autism' (rather than the less specific form of ASD). Mikita et al. (unpublished) found no relationship between the presence of high irritability and any of the domains of the autism spectrum.

Alternatively, irritability might reflect a general problem in coping with the challenges of the world. This, however, was made unlikely by the finding from Simonoff et al. (2012) that neither IQ nor adaptive function discriminated ASD subjects from controls.

Affected children might not understand other people's reactions, and misinterpret them as threatening. The ability to recognize emotions in other people's faces was indeed worse in the irritable 16-year-olds tested by Simonoff et al. (2012) than in their controls (with autism but no severe mood problem). Full interpretation of this finding is difficult. It stemmed largely from children's difficulty in recognizing the emotion of surprise, not that of anger. However, it was not attributable to a generally low IQ, since the finding also emerged when only those with an IQ higher than 70 were analysed. Limited understanding can also be responsible for paranoid beliefs about the malicious intentions of other people. A few young people may harbour deep-seated resentment about individuals, such as siblings who are perceived as being favoured, to the extent that they become dangerous towards them.

Affected children might have less cognitive flexibility, and therefore be more susceptible to anger arousal, as suggested in Chapter 6. The Wisconsin Card Sorting Test, applied by Simonoff et al, (2012), did suggest that the 'severe mood problem' group differed from other children with ASD in this way. Interpretation is somewhat uncertain, as the apparent result was no longer significant when IQ was controlled for—but this does not necessarily invalidate the finding. (It might for instance apply only in the presence of low IQ.)

Affected children might have an altered reaction to stress. This idea was explored by Mikita et al. (unpublished) in their physiological study of children and adolescents with high-functioning autism. Within this group, irritable children (as identified by themselves) were likely to have a lower cortisol response to stress and also (as identified by parents) to have a lower heart rate response. This could parallel the low physiological reactivity to stress that was reported for boys with ODD who were not on the autism spectrum (van Goozen et al., 1998). Indeed, anxiety played a role in the findings of Mikita and colleagues, and they may not be very specific to irritability. Nevertheless, the finding of low reactivity adds some weight to the notion that states of irritability and mood disturbance are not simply part of the autism spectrum but represent an additional and separate problem.

High irritability might be a function of the other mental disorders to which children in the autism spectrum are prone. For example, Bradley et al. (2006) described episodic emotional disorders in 17/36 children with autism and learning disorder and found them to be more common than in learning disorder alone. Only two of these 17 children were diagnosed with bipolar disorder—the others had a mixture of diagnoses, with the most common being depression. Irritability, however, was not specifically studied in this investigation.

Simonoff et al. (2012) did, however, find that children in their 'severe mood problem' group were much more likely than other children with ASD to have a parent with an affective disorder. Furthermore, this was not due to the burden of care that falls on the parents of children with autism. A measure of parenting stress did not show a difference for the families where the children had major problems of angry and miserable mood. This is similar to the findings of depression in family members, both in the Bradley and Bolton study (Bradley et al., 2006) and in children with SMD who do not have an ASD (Brotman et al., 2007).

In the Simonoff et al. study of severe mood problems, no one coexistent condition was more common in the group with severe mood problems than in their controls, not even depression; but there was a strong relationship with the number of coexistent conditions. The likelihood of severe mood problems varied from 3% with no other diagnosis than ASD, to 32% with one other diagnosis, and to 44% for those with two or more other diagnoses.

The irritability of some young people with autism might reflect a transactional process, in which the trouble they give to their caregivers elicits angry and threatening responses, to which their own response is angry and sometimes aggressive. This developmental path would be in keeping with a similar progression proposed for ADHD in Chapter 7. We have not found any investigations that tested this possibility directly. Nevertheless, clinicians should bear in mind the possibility of harsh treatment and assess accordingly.

In summary, research has not established the developmental pathways involved in the associations between ASD and outbursts of anger, and still less to dysphoric states. There are many gaps in knowledge that will need filling: not only with larger numbers of subjects in the case–control paradigms described but also with methods giving longitudinal information on trajectories, and with applications of genetically informative designs and neurophysiological and cognitive measures. At this early stage of knowledge we consider that the main lessons for clinicians are:

♦ Dysphoric states involving irritability are not an integral part of autism, but need separate recognition and management.

♦ Irritability is linked to miserable mood in ASD as in typically developing children.

♦ Irritability can and should be reliably assessed, and the methods outlined in Chapter 3 are suitable even in the presence of ASD.

Management of irritability in people with ASD

It is easy for mood changes in ASD to be overshadowed by the ASD diagnosis and therefore not be given their full weight in treatment planning. Detection of the mood problem of irritability is helped by the use of screening questionnaires, as considered in Chapter 3. The Aberrant Behavior Checklist (ABC; Aman et al., 1985) contains an irritability subscale (ABC-I). It consists of 16 items, including self-injurious behaviours, physical aggression towards others, screaming, yelling, temper tantrums, demanding behaviours, mood changes, and crying in response to minor annoyances. This is perhaps not specifically a measure of 'irritability', but includes many 'oppositional defiant' problems too. The Overt Aggression Scale-Modified (OAS-M; Yudofsky et al., 1986), the Child Autism Rating Scale (CARS; Schopler et al., 1986), and the Affective Reactivity Index (ARI; Stringaris et al., 2012a) (see Chapter 3 and the Apppendix) are also appropriate for use in this group.

Detailed accounts of the problems should be taken from parents, teachers, and when possible from the young people themselves. The parental account is particularly useful for establishing the course of problems over time, the situations at home that elicit outbursts, and the young person's usual mood state in everyday situations. The account from school is particularly helpful for understanding any situational specificity and the level of impairment that can be attributed to irritability. The account from the child or adolescent is particularly informative for understanding their mood states and their understanding of what or who is responsible for their angry feelings.

A functional analysis aims to determine what the irritability is achieving. The accounts of problems may be clear enough to allow the clinician to determine the functions for the individual child in terms of when anger appears, which situations provoke it, how it is expressed, and what its consequences are. Angry outbursts may, for instance, be seen to be signalling unmet need. Painful conditions such as toothache, earache, and constipation may be creating both the distress involved and the frustration of being unable to express the need to caregivers. Often, however, it is necessary to observe the child for periods of an hour or more in different natural settings.

Psychological treatments

Such an analysis leads naturally to a treatment plan, to be discussed with all concerned. 'Positive behaviour support' follows functional analysis with a plan to teach adaptive skills—often in the ability to communicate—that can replace the tantrums or aggression that are distressing (Carr et al., 2002). Details will of course vary with the individual.

A psychosocial treatment programme along these lines was evaluated by Aman et al. (2009) in a randomized controlled trial, comparing it (given together with medication) with medication as the only intervention, in a group of 124 children aged 9 to 13 who showed a combination of 'pervasive developmental disorder' and behavioural problems such as tantrums, aggression, and self-injury. It trained parents and children in a series of individual sessions, focusing on the development of communication, appropriate use of rewards, encouragement of compliance, and learning adaptive skills. The treatment was not aimed specifically at irritability, but ABC-I was one of the outcome measures. Behavioural problems did decrease, and irritability in particular was substantially reduced, with a substantial effect size of 0.48 by comparison with the medication-only group.

Developing an autism-friendly environment is also an important part of educating the children. Some of the measures involved are intended to reduce the distressing and disruptive effects of anger outbursts. The triggers to anger can be reduced by ensuring a high degree of structure and order, so that children can have clear expectations of what they will be doing, where, and when. Calmness in the people looking after them prevents escalating cycles of aggression, and calls for careful support of the caregivers and teachers.

Pharmacotherapies

Pharmacological treatment has been evaluated in a series of randomized controlled trials comparing drugs and placebo. Several well-controlled studies have been carried out under the auspices of the Research Units on

Pediatric Psychopharmacology (RUPP) Autism Network. Irritability is either the primary outcome or one of the secondary outcomes in several of the trials. Systematic reviews are provided in Canitano et al. (2011) and Elbe et al. (2012).

Risperidone is the best-evaluated of the drugs. It is an antipsychotic agent that antagonizes dopaminergic transmission at the synapse between nerve cells. Typically it is given in rather low dosage: in the trial by Aman et al. (2009), the daily dose for children weighing less than 20 kg was 0.25–1.75 mg; for those weighing 20–45 kg it was 0.5–2.5 mg; and for those weighing more than 45 kg it was 0.5–3.5 mg. Several randomized controlled trials have compared risperidone with placebo in people with ASD; they are summarized separately in Box 8.2 in view of the controversy surrounding this indication.

Longer-term effects were described by Zuddas et al. (2000) and Aman et al. (2005). Troost et al. (2005) reported a double-blind trial in a group of 24 children, all of whom were short-term responders. After 24 weeks they either switched to placebo or persisted with the risperidone; there was continued efficacy for about half of the cases.

Box 8.2 Risperidone trials

♦ RUPPAN (2002) treated 101 children aged 5 to 17 years. The ABC-I declined by some 15 points with the active treatment but only 3.6 on placebo.

♦ Shea et al. (2004) treated 79 children with a mean age around 7.6 years. The ABC-I declined by 12 points in the treated group but only 6.5 points in those given placebo.

♦ Hellings et al. (2006) treated 40 people aged from 8 to 56 years. The ABC-I declined by 8 points in the treated group and 6.5 points with placebo.

♦ Nagaraj et al. (2006) treated 39 children with a mean age of 4.8 years. On the CARS the active treatment group reduced by 7.5 points and placebo by 1.0.

♦ Luby et al. (2006) treated 23 children with a mean age around 4 years. On the CARS the active treatment group declined by 4.6 points and placebo by 1.8.

♦ Pandina et al. (2007) treated 55 children, mean around 7 years. The ABC-I declined in the treated group by 13.4 points and placebo by 7.5.

Aripiprazole was evaluated by Owen et al.(2009) for 98 children and Marcus et al. (2009) for 218. In both these randomized trials, the ABC-I showed a greater reduction by the active drug than by a placebo, and the size of the action was comparable to that of risperidone.

Olanzapine was compared with placebo by Hollander et al. (2006) in a randomized controlled trial conducted on a small group of 11 children: the result for irritability was substantial (but so were the effects on weight gain).

In summary, every trial that has competently assessed the effects of low doses of antipsychotics on scales measuring broad aspects of irritability has found their efficacy to be significant, and to endure over periods of several months. The drugs may well be acting in a non-specific way, to reduce anxiety and aggression; and they do not of course make a substantial difference to the core symptoms of autism.

The other side of the equation is the adverse effects of these drugs. These are not specific to autism but apply across the whole range of indications for which they are given and are described more fully in Chapter 14. Obesity is very common, and sedation and endocrine and metabolic abnormalities can also be seen. De Hert et al. (2011) reviewed 24 trials of risperidone in children and adolescents. Not all were in children with autism, but there was a trend for children with autism to have more problems with the drug than others, perhaps because they were in general being treated at an earlier age. There were more than 3000 children in the studies, and they had a strong tendency to undue weight gain, hyperprolactinaemia, and associated metabolic disturbances.

The adverse effects of the drugs can be lasting. In a 48-week open trial, risperidone (mean dose 1.5 mg) had continuing effects on weight gain as well as continued efficacy in controlling disruptive behaviour (Findling et al., 2004). Weight gain at a level judged to be an adverse event affected 21% of 107 children aged 5 to 12 who were being treated for disruptive behaviour disorders in the context of subaverage intelligence. The mean weight gain was 5.5 kg, which was at least twice that expected. In other respects the drug was reasonably well tolerated over this extended period. The risk of obesity and metabolic problems is greater in those who are already overweight or have a family history of diabetes. Careful monitoring is essential (see Chapter 14). Clinicians should be alert to the possibility of subtle effects on blunting cognition.

Aripiprazole has a reputation for being less hazardous, but in the Marcus et al. (2009) trial over an 8-week period the treated children, even on the low dose of 5 mg, had gained an average of 1.3 kg in weight. In the Owen et al. (2009) trial the mean weight gain was 2.0 kg on aripiprazole (variable dose) and 0.8 kg on placebo over an 8-week period. Metabolic abnormalities were not, however, noted in these rather short trials.

Clinicians must balance the risks against the possible gains on an individual basis. There is a favourable balance of benefit over risk in severe cases—where irritability is hampering the individual's development—for periods up to about 6 months, and regulatory agencies have correspondingly licensed risperidone for severe irritability in autism (Morgan et al., 2007).

It has been natural to seek other medications with less risk. Small-scale pilot studies with randomization have found promising reductions in the irritability of children in the autism spectrum with divalproex sodium (55 children, mean age 9.5 years; Hollander et al., 2010) and N-acetylcysteine (33 children, age 3 to 12; Hardan et al., 2012). These do not, however, constitute a sufficient evidence base to establish them as anything but alternative therapies. They should therefore be reserved for specific indications and when other treatments have failed or are contraindicated, and when consent has been accordingly informed. Methylphenidate does not appear to be useful unless ADHD is also present—in which case it is a safer alternative and should probably be tried first (Simonoff et al., 2012) (see Chapter 7).

Chapter 9

Irritability and disruptive behaviour disorders

Oppositional–defiant disorder (ODD) describes an enduring trait of developmentally inappropriate and impairing problems of non-compliant behaviour and negative mood. Irritability is part of the definition.

DSM-5 describes ODD as a common condition involving both behaviour problems and negative mood. Anger, resentment, and easily becoming annoyed all represent irritability: three such symptoms enter into the diagnostic criteria, together with four of headstrong, non-compliant, and defiant behaviour and one of vindictiveness; diagnostic criteria are said to be met if four out of the possible eight are present.

Most children with ODD will, by definition, show irritability too. Nevertheless, the irritable component can and should be distinguished from others. Recently, Stringaris and Goodman (Stringaris et al., 2009d) proposed three distinct dimensions within oppositionality: an irritable dimension that predicts primarily depressive disorders and generalized anxiety disorder; a headstrong dimension related to ADHD and non-aggressive conduct disorder (CD); and a hurtful dimension associated with aggressive conduct problems and callous/unemotional traits. The differential associations of the three dimensions of ODD have been demonstrated in cross-sectional and longitudinal community-based samples (Stringaris et al., 2009b; Aebi et al., 2010; Rowe et al., 2010; Krieger et al., 2013).

In Chapter 5 we emphasized the developmental differences between these components of ODD. At the level of current symptoms, factor analysis has supported the distinction; analysis of longitudinal data sets has indicated the specific link between irritability and later depression (Stringaris et al., 2009b). Rowe et al. (2010) and Burke et al. (2010) have reported a similar link. Drabick and Gadow (Drabick et al., 2012) were able to separate two distinct groups of children with ODD: one with angry/irritable features and one with non-compliant behaviours who did not meet the angry/irritable criteria. The irritable group was characterized by a high rate of other emotional problems (anxiety and depression). Conversely, Speltz et al. (1999) focused on children with both ODD and emotional problems. In comparison with children with ODD who did not have emotional problems, their profile of ODD symptoms was more likely to include irritability items: touchy/easily annoyed, angry/resentful, and spiteful/vindictive.

This strong link between irritability and depression is taken further in Chapter 10, on depression.

Prevalence and comorbidity

ODD is common in the population at large: a systematic review of epidemiological studies by Boylan et al. (2007) found most estimates to converge on a range of 3–6% for young people of school age. A higher rate, of up to 12%, is often described in preschool children (Lavigne et al., 2001). It is one of the commonest diagnoses in child mental health clinics—accounting for 28–65% of diagnoses in different surveys (Boylan et al., 2007), with the higher figures being drawn from clinics dealing specifically with behavioural problems.

Estimates of prevalence are subject to many difficulties. The defining problems can, individually, all be part of typical child development (Chapter 4). The distinctive feature of ODD is one of degree. The apparent frequency therefore depends on setting a cut-off, and including impairment in the definition; both of which have to proceed without definitive scientific evidence about where the cut-off should be placed and how impairment should be defined. The apparently high rates in preschool children, and their variation between studies, may well reflect particular uncertainty about the nature of impairment at this age. Adult tolerance and competence may have a strong role in the construction of a 'disorder'.

Association with conduct disorder

Categorical diagnostic schemes struggle to achieve clarity in the delineation of ODD (including irritability) from other disruptive disorders (and see Fig.14.1 and the accompanying text in Chapter 14 for an attempt to provide a guide to the confusing welter of overlapping categories).

The DSM-5 and ICD-10 schemes take different approaches. In DSM-5, ODD is separate from, but can coexist with, 'conduct disorder', in which antisocial behaviour is severe enough to be violating the basic rights of others but in which mood problems play no part in the diagnostic criteria.

ICD-10 also describes ODD as a very common condition, and uses very similar criteria to those of the DSM, but treats comorbidity in a different way. ODD is regarded as a milder and earlier form of CD, and is not diagnosed if the antisocial behaviour problems have reached the level of CD.

This controversy about the relationship between ODD and CD has generated substantial research, especially from longitudinal studies about their developmental relationship. Certainly ODD is typically present before CD begins, and ODD is a significant predictor of whether CD will develop; many adolescents with CD have an earlier story of ODD (Lahey et al., 1992). Nevertheless, they are not identical. The well-known Great Smoky Mountains Study of Youth (Costello et al., 1996) is a longitudinal, epidemiologically based study with over 8000 observations on 1420 individuals between the ages of 9 and 21 years. It reported significant prediction from ODD to CD, but by no means a direct continuity (Rowe et al., 2010). Most of those with ODD did not develop CD. CD arising for the first time in adolescence did not have a direct link with earlier ODD. CD did not have specific associations with emotional disorders, unlike the case for the irritable component of ODD.

Association with ADHD

ODD is also very common in people with ADHD, especially if impulsiveness is a prominent part of the ADHD, to the extent that researchers of ADHD often do not report ODD as a comorbidity at all, considering it as a key part of the condition.

The 'comorbidity' with ADHD is dealt with differently in ICD and DSM. In ICD-10, the equivalent category is 'hyperkinetic disorder', which is based on the same symptoms as ADHD but requires more of them, and more pervasiveness, for the diagnosis. When it coexists with disruptive behaviour, then

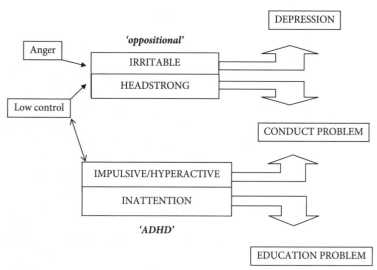

Fig. 9.1 A simplified way of formulating the developmental progress of oppositional and irritable children.

the diagnosis is 'hyperkinetic conduct disorder', reflecting the evidence that the comorbid condition carries the same neurodevelopmental and therapeutic implications as does hyperkinetic disorder alone.

We find it clinically helpful to conceptualize these closely related conditions as comprising four dimensional components, as set out in Fig. 9.1: irritability, non-compliance, impulsiveness (with overactivity), and inattention. They often coexist, but have different developmental implications. The impulsiveness of ADHD includes the element of poor behavioural control, which influences non-compliant behaviour, and both predict to antisocial behaviour (including CD) later.

Management

For the clinician, the implication of this is that a single diagnosis of ODD, ADHD, or CD is not usually a sufficient guide to practice. Rather, each component should be considered for its severity and its impact upon the child's functioning. The social influences on whether ODD develops (Chapter 4), and whether it is presented as a problem, imply that they need to be considered, as much as intra-individual pathology.

The irritability component is to be recognized by the principles of Chapter 3, and managed along the lines of Chapter 14. When another, treatable diagnosis is present—such as ADHD, depression, bipolar disorder, or challenging behaviour in ASD/autism—then that will probably take precedence in therapeutic planning (see previous chapters). A review of case progress should then consider whether ODD traits are present even at times when the primary diagnosis is in remission or controlled. When that is the case, the generic approaches—particularly parenting interventions that have an evidence base for treating ODD—described in Chapter 14 need to be applied. DMDD, however, includes the symptoms of ODD at a higher level of severity, so it is not appropriate here to recognize ODD separately.

The antisocial problems of CD make the assessment of risks to others particularly germane. Is there evidence of previous dangerous behaviour? Is there any person who is particularly at risk? Have there been threats and menaces to other people? Is there misuse of alcohol, illegal substances, or so-called recreational highs that might potentiate violence? Are there any social circumstances likely to magnify the risk of violence, such as gang membership? None of these are specific to irritability, but they may be occurring in people whose irritability has contributed to bringing them into a high-risk category. Confidentiality will need to be breached if they divulge intentions of harm to others, or indeed to themselves, so absolute assurance of confidentiality should not be given.

Chapter 10

Irritability and bipolar disorder

Irritability is not a problem 'associated with' bipolar disorder: it is an essential part of the definition. An intense debate surrounds the concept of bipolar disorder in children. Irritability is at the heart of the problem. It is often present in depression (see Chapter 11) and is a defining feature of mania (along with euphoria and grandiosity and the presence of associated features such as a decreased need for sleep, over-talkativeness, and an abnormally high level of distractibility and/or activities that are pleasurable but likely to have adverse consequences).

On the one hand, irritability is regarded by some national guidelines as a non-specific problem, often present in mania but insufficient in itself to establish the diagnosis (NICE, 2006). On the other hand, some authorities teach that mania in children often presents as irritability, and that irritability is a sufficient mood change (in combination with associated features) for a diagnosis of mania (Wozniak et al., 1995).

An episodic nature and chronicity are also crucial to the debate. While traditional psychiatric thinking defines bipolarity as consisting of distinct episodes of mood disturbance, sometimes depressive and sometimes manic—as in the DSM-5 descriptions (American Psychiatric Association, 2013)—many authorities consider that the condition in children and adolescents can be chronic, with manic and depressive features often existing in a persistent and non-episodic way, and term it 'paediatric bipolar disorder' (Spencer et al., 2001).

This argument has great practical implications. Over the last 15 years, the rates of diagnosis of bipolar disorder in children and adolescents in the United States have increased dramatically, in both in-patient (Blader et al., 2007) and out-patient services (Moreno et al., 2007). The increase in rates of bipolar diagnoses occurred in parallel with a rise in prescription rates for antipsychotic medication (Olfson et al., 2006). Diagnostic practice seems to be the most likely explanation for the observed increase in bipolar diagnoses (Leibenluft, 2011).

Confusion therefore exists in the literature, and it is not always easy to discern which concept is being used by the authors and therefore how to translate this into clinical practice. In this chapter, for clarity, we shall make a distinction. We first describe the role of irritability in the DSM-5 type of episodic bipolar disorder, and its management. We then contrast it with the mood change of severe and chronic dysregulation. This has been called by some 'paediatric bipolar disorder', but we prefer not to use that term as it has not yet been shown that chronic mood dysregulation is in fact a variant of bipolar disorder as usually defined. The arguments about defining bipolar disorder are complex and require further empirical work (Stringaris, 2011). The chapter concludes with consideration of a grey area between these formulations. Suffice it to say that the claim that chronic irritability may be a pathognomonic feature of bipolar disorder in young people—the 'paediatric bipolar disorder' phenotype—has very little evidence in its favour. Indeed, a follow-up study has shown that manic episodes are extremely rare among children with severe chronic irritability (Stringaris et al., 2010a).

First, however, we shall describe how the apparent prevalence of bipolar disorder in the child and adolescent population has changed over time; because this illustrates the complexities of the diagnostic enterprise.

Epidemiological data on the prevalence of bipolar disorder in children and adolescents

Bipolar disorder in children has traditionally been thought to be rare (Goodwin et al., 2007) and epidemiological data are consistent with this view.

The Great Smoky Mountains Study of Youth used a multistage overlapping cohorts design to study a random sample of 1015 children in the southeastern United States (Costello et al., 1996). The authors established DSM-III-R diagnoses using an interview-based measure, the Child and Adolescent Psychiatric Assessment (CAPA) (Angold et al., 1995a,b). They found that the 3-month prevalence of mania was 0 and that the 3-month prevalence of hypomania was $0.1 \pm 0.06\%$ (Costello et al., 1996). This is a very small estimate compared with some examples of the main anxiety disorders: the 3-month prevalence for separation anxiety disorder is $3.49\% \pm 0.75$ and for generalized anxiety disorder $1.67\% \pm 0.61$.

Lewinsohn et al. (1993) ascertained DSM-III-R diagnoses in adolescents from nine high schools (Grades 9–12) in a mixture of urban and rural communities in Oregon, United States. The young people were interviewed twice, at a mean age of 16.6 years (Time 1) and a year later (Time 2), using a semi-structured interview, K-SADS (Chambers et al., 1985) to ascertain DSM-III-R diagnoses. They found that the lifetime prevalence of bipolar disorder was $0.58 \pm 0.18\%$ at Time 1 and $0.66 \pm 0.21\%$ at Time 2. This is a very small estimate compared, for example, with that for unipolar depression, where the lifetime prevalence was $20.35 \pm 0.97\%$ at Time 1 and $25.27 \pm 1.12\%$ at Time 2.

A study by Stringaris et al. (2010b) used the 2004 British Child and Adolescent Mental Health Survey (B-CAMHS04) with data on a representative sample of 5326 children aged between 8 and 19 years. The authors used the Development and Wellbeing Assessment (DAWBA), a structured interview administered by lay interviewers; its questions are closely related to the DSM-IV criteria (American Psychiatric Association, 2000) and focus on current, rather than lifetime, problems (Goodman et al., 2000; Ford et al., 2003). Stringaris et al. (2010b) found that only seven individuals (0.1%) met either probable or definite DSM-IV criteria for bipolar disorder I or II.

It perhaps also says something important about the expectations of continental European child psychiatrists concerning the prevalence of bipolar disorder that several landmark epidemiological studies have decided against ascertaining bipolar disorder as a diagnostic outcome (Esser et al., 1990; Fombonne, 1994; Steinhausen et al., 1998; Wittchen et al., 1998).

The rise in diagnostic rates of bipolar disorder in children and adolescents

This status of bipolar disorder as a rarity among young people was challenged by a dramatic increase in its diagnosis over the past decade in data from US psychiatric clinics and in-patient settings.

Blader and Carlson used data from the National Hospital Discharge Survey (NHDS) to study the rates of bipolar diagnoses among US youth and adults admitted as in-patients between 1996 and 2004 (Blader et al., 2007). Using a probability sample of hospitals, the NHDS documents anonymized patient-level discharge information. Single individuals may be represented more than once (e.g. if they have been discharged twice from a hospital that was sampled twice) and therefore the estimates presented in the paper do not reflect individuals but discharges. The authors identified discharges associated with a psychiatric disorder by extracting ICD-based (ICD-9-CM) diagnoses which are, according to the authors (NCHS, 2006), congruent with DSM-IV (American Psychiatric Association, 2000).

The authors found that psychiatrically related discharges from hospital grew considerably overall, particularly for the younger ages. Among children (age range 5–13 years) the increase between 1996 and 2004 was 53.2%, for adolescents (ages 14–18) the increase was 58.5%, and for adults (anyone aged over 18 years) only 3.3%. Against this background of increasing discharges, the authors found that the proportion of discharges with a diagnosis of bipolar disorder rose dramatically. As a proportion of the total number of psychiatrically related discharges, children with diagnoses of bipolar disorder constituted 10% in 1996 and 34.11% in 2004. The figures for adolescents were 10.24% and 25.86% for 1996 and 2004, respectively. For adults, bipolar disorder as a proportion of the total number of psychiatrically related discharges was 9.9% in 1996 and 14.9% in 2004. The authors also found that the change in the US rates for groups of psychiatric disorders appearing as primary diagnoses for acute care in-patients from 1996 to 2004 was dramatically higher for the diagnosis of bipolar disorder in young people—children in particular—compared with adults and with any other diagnostic group. Fig. 10.1 depicts this increase, with data extracted from Table 1 of Blader et al. (2007, p. 110) (change is expressed as the difference between 2004 rates per 10 000 minus 1996 rates divided by the 1996 figure).

Blader and Carlson (Blader et al., 2007; Moreno et al., 2007) discuss several possible explanations for what could have accounted for such a dramatic increase in bipolar disorder discharge diagnoses, especially among children. Of the various possibilities, they seem to favour the explanation that:

> . . . , growth in the rate of BD-diagnosed discharges might reflect a progressive "rebranding" of the same clinical phenomena for which hospitalized children previously received different diagnoses. The unchanged rate of conduct problem diagnoses over survey years represents an effective decline in light of the marked rise in overall population-adjusted rate of children's psychiatric discharges. Clinicians may have responded to the higher hurdles of obtaining payers' authorization for inpatient care by "upcoding" severe behavioral disturbances to a major mood disorder that connotes a more pernicious illness. (Blader et al., 2007, p. 112).

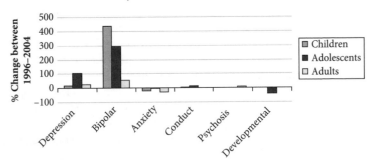

Changes in US Rates for Groups of Psychiatric Disorders Coded as Primary Diagnoses in Acute US Inpatient Units from 1996–2004 (source: Blader and Carlson 2007)

Fig. 10.1 Changes in US in-patient diagnoses.

Reprinted from Biological Psychiatry, 62, Blader, J. C., et al, Increased rates of bipolar disorder diagnoses among U.S. child, adolescent, and adult inpatients, 1996–2004, 107, Copyright (2007), with permission from Elsevier.

The authors continue by noting the differences in sex ratios in their data where:

> male children outnumber females while among adults females predominate hint[ing] at a different disorder (Blader et al., 2007, p 113).

Moreno et al. (2007) conducted a study using the National Ambulatory Medical Care Survey (NAMCS) to study the national trends of diagnoses of bipolar disorder in children in the United States compared with adults between the years 1999 and 2003. The NAMCS is conducted annually in the United States by the National Center for Health Statistics. It samples a 'nationally representative group of visits to non-federally employed office-based physicians who are primarily engaged in direct patient care' (Moreno et al., 2007, p. 1033), using a probability sample design. During one given week, physicians or their office staff complete a one-page document to gather demographic clinical and treatment characteristics of their patients. Diagnoses were made by the treating physicians according to ICD-9-CM (NCHS, 2006).

As illustrated in Fig. 10.2, constructed from data given on p. 1034 of the paper by Moreno et al. (2007), the rise in the rate of bipolar diagnoses expressed as a percentage of total office-based visits was much sharper for young people (age range 0–19) than for adults (aged ≥ 20 years). The difference in increase was significant as evidenced by the significant age group and year interaction.

Moreno et al. (2007) also found that young people coded as suffering from bipolar disorder visits were considerably more likely to be male (66.5%) than were the adults with a diagnosis of bipolar disorder, who were predominantly female (67.6%). In addition, young people were 10 times more likely to

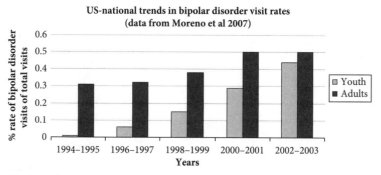

Fig. 10.2 Changes in US out-patient diagnoses.

Data from Moreno et al (2007).

receive a comorbid diagnosis of ADHD than were adults (32.2% compared with 3.0%). Finally, the authors also report that young people (90.6%) were as likely as were adults (86.4%) to receive psychotropic medication during bipolar visits, with comparable rates of mood stabilizers, antipsychotics, and antidepressants for both groups.

Moreno et al. (2007) consider two main possible explanations for their findings. First, that the sharp increase in bipolar diagnoses in young people could be accounted for by increased recognition of the condition by treating physicians, perhaps partly attributable to attention that has been drawn to the condition by the mass media (Moreno et al., 2007, p. 1036). Alternatively, they consider the possibility that the increases are due to over-diagnosis of bipolar disorder in young people and suggest that overlap between ADHD and paediatric bipolar disorder may be an important source of 'diagnostic uncertainty' (Moreno et al., 2007, p. 1036). One of their conclusions is that:

> Our analyses suggest that boys with comorbid ADHD may account for the pre-dominance of males among youth diagnosed with bipolar disorder. Without prospective longitudinal research, it is not possible to determine the extent to which pediatric bipolar disorder is a developmental subtype of the adult illness characterized by this sex and comorbidity pattern or the extent to which *highly irritable boys with ADHD* [emphasis added] are being misdiagnosed as having bipolar disorder. (Moreno et al., 2007, p. 1037)

Concurrent with this increase in diagnoses of bipolar disorder was a rise in prescription rates for antipsychotic medication for children and adolescents, as measured using the NAMCS data (Olfson et al., 2006). In Fig. 10.3,

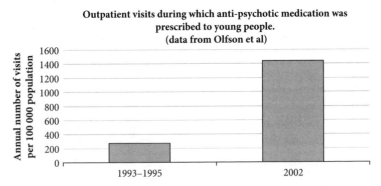

Outpatient visits during which anti-psychotic medication was prescribed to young people.
(data from Olfson et al)

Fig. 10.3 Changes to prescription rates of antipsychotic medication for young people.

Data from Olfson et al (2006).

data extracted from that paper depict the rise in antipsychotic medication prescribed to young people (age range 0–21 years) during outpatient visits to physicians. Olfson et al. (2006) found that the linear trend for these data was statistically significant. They also found that:

> Among young mental health visits that included a prescription of an anti-psychotic medication, disruptive behavior disorders (37.8%) and mood disorders (31.8%) tended to be more frequently diagnosed than pervasive developmental disorders (17.3%) or mental retardation (17.3%) or psychotic disorders (14.2%). . . . (Olfson et al., 2006, p. 682)

Interestingly, in approximately a third of those visits where antipsychotics were prescribed a co-prescription of antidepressants was made; in addition, a third of visits where antipsychotics were prescribed included a co-prescription of mood-stabilizing medication (Olfson et al., 2006).

This rise in the apparent prevalence in the United States over time illustrates the need for clarity in diagnosis, and its importance in decisions about treatment.

Irritability in episodic bipolar disorder

The DSM-5 criteria for bipolar disorder specify the need for a 'distinct period of abnormally and persistently elevated, expansive or irritable mood'. In contrast to the criteria for major depressive episodes, the criteria for manic episodes and bipolar disorder do not differ between children and adults in either DSM-5 or ICD-10. DSM-5 provides that irritability can be the predominant mood of a manic episode even if unaccompanied by the other mood changes. (This is in contrast to the practice in other countries, including England and Wales, where advice from the National Institute for Health and Care Excellence is that irritability without elation or grandiosity should not allow a diagnosis of mania in children; NICE, 2006.)

This mood should be accompanied by three or more symptoms (or four if only irritability is present)[1] that are characteristic of mania, such as grandiosity or a flight of ideas that occur at the same time as the episodic change in mood. The duration of the episode is expected to be at least a week for bipolar I, but may be as short as four days for an episode of hypomania (and a diagnosis of bipolar II).

---

[1] This requirement for four, as opposed to the usual three, symptoms when the mood is irritable may be seen as implicit recognition of the fact that irritability is less pathognomonic than euphoria and grandiosity, and that this lower specificity therefore needs to be balanced by more additional features.

Management of manic states

For the irritability of the manic state itself, careful and calm explanation is needed for the family as well as the patient: it will often be a first episode, and therefore all the more frightening. Establishing a therapeutic relationship needs to be a priority from the first contact. There will be difficult decisions to make about therapy, and the condition is likely to recur. The safety of the young person and others needs to be addressed. The ability of the family to manage the risks should be judged; urgent admission to an in-patient unit is often wise because of the inherent unpredictability of the person's mental state.

The drugs widely used for acute treatment of mania in adult psychiatry— lithium, antiepileptic drugs, and antipsychotics—are often employed for children who are affected. Guidelines, for example from United States and England and Wales, recommend their use in young people (McClellan et al., 2007). There have, however, been only a few double-blind randomized controlled trials of drug treatments in this age group. Several systematic reviews have been undertaken (e.g. Consoli et al., 2007; Correll et al., 2010; Liu et al., 2011); a meta-analysis of adult data by Cipriani et al. (2011) is also relevant. The trials do not take irritability as a target symptom: the usual outcome measure is the Young Mania Rating Scale which includes items both of irritability and other features of mania; but irritability is very commonly present during episodes of mania in children and adolescents. For an overview of treatment of manic states please also refer to the relevant chapter of the latest Maudsley Prescrbing Guidelines (Zahreddine and Stringaris 2014).

Antipsychotics

Antipsychotic medications and their actions are described in Chapter 14. A few studies have compared their actions with placebo or with antipsychotics in children and adolescents.

In two randomized controlled trials of aripiprazole it was superior to placebo. Findling et al. (2009) found a positive response in 16/18 youngsters given aripiprazole but only 13/25 for placebo. Tramontino et al. (2009) found a similar superiority, achieving a positive response in 44/98 compared with 26/99 on placebo.

A randomized controlled trial of risperidone against placebo found a positive response in 29/50 given the drug but in only 15/58 receiving placebo (Haas et al., 2009).

Tohen et al. (2007) found that olanzapine was superior to placebo in a trial including 161 adolescents, with response rates of 44.8% in the active treatment group and 18.5% in the comparator group. A price was paid, however; there was a high rate of weight gain and metabolic alterations in the olanzapine-treated group.

Quetiapine is effective for the treatment of mania in young people with bipolar disorder Type I (Pathak et al 2013).

Open studies of antipsychotics in the short term have also been reported. Olanzapine was associated with a good outcome in 50% of youngsters (Frazier et al., 2001). Risperidone achieved response rates of 82.4% in combination with lithium and 80% in combination with divalproate (Pavuluri et al., 2004). Another series reported naturalistic response rates of risperidone and olanzapine at around 70% (Biederman et al., 2005). Ziprasidone, too, has been described, with 57% of recipients regarded as responders (Biederman et al., 2007), and aripiprazole with 67% (Barzman et al., 2004). Even clozapine (with particularly worrying adverse effects extending to blood cell formation as well as sugar and lipid metabolism) has some report of value (Masi et al., 2002).

The adverse effects of antipsychotics, and the choice of drug, are considered in Chapter 14. These effects are substantial, especially in the longer term. However, for the acute and short-term treatment of mania antipsychotics are superior to the other available medicines.

Antiepileptics

Out of four trials of mood stabilizers in children and adolescents reviewed by Correll et al. (2010) only one showed a significant superiority to placebo.

Several observational studies had previously reported modestly encouraging results. Response rates for divalproex alone were reported at 67% (Deltito et al., 1998) and 61% (Wagner et al., 2002). In a study reporting a series of young people treated with various mood stabilizers, there were response rates of 38% for lithium, 53% for divalproate, and 38% for carbamazepine (Kowatch et al., 2003). Henry et al. (2003) made a chart review of the longer-term outcome in young people: 8 out of 15 were judged to have made a moderate or good response.

Lithium

Lithium has well-established indications in adults for prophylaxis of mania and potentiation of antidepressant drugs. It has multiple actions on membrane function and neurotransmitters (Jope, 1999). For children, there are uncertainties about efficacy, there can be problems in the need for close monitoring of blood levels and thyroid and kidney function, and there is a high rate of adverse events in young children (Hagino et al., 1995). The therapeutic level in the blood should be in the range between 0.8 and 1.2 mmol/l. There is, however, little evidence that lithium is efficacious at all in the treatment of acute mania in young people (Liu et al., 2011).

In various open trials of acute treatment, response rates for lithium alone have been reported as 63% by Kafantaris et al. (2003); 68% and 80.6% in the absence of ADHD but 57.7% in its presence (Strober et al., 1998); and 42% for a combination of lithium and divalproate (Findling et al., 2003). These studies have several limitations: not only the lack of control procedures but also the sometimes small numbers, short duration (up to 8 weeks), uncertainty over subject descriptions, and lack of standard outcome criteria.

Antipsychotics versus mood stabilizers

Antipsychotics are more efficacious in the short term than mood stabilizers. Correll et al. (2010) made a systematic comparison of effect sizes in five trials of antipsychotics and four of lithium or antiepileptics in young people. There was a substantial superiority for antipsychotics (0.68 SD). There was also a higher risk for adverse effects. Head-to-head trials have told a similar story.

Liu et al. (2011) randomly assigned 279 6- to 15-year-old patients to receive lithium, divalproex sodium, or risperidone: lithium and valproex were less efficacious than risperidone but had fewer adverse effects on weight gain and prolactin. In the absence of a placebo control, it is not possible to tell whether the smaller effect of the mood stabilizers would have been therapeutically useful.

Pavuluri et al. (2010) randomly assigned 66 young people (mean age about 10 years) to either risperidone or valproex. The response rate on the Young Mania Rating Scale was 78.1% for risperidone but only 45.5% for divalproex. Safety measures were similar for both, but more children dropped out if they had been assigned to valproex, largely because of an increase in irritability.

Clinical recommendations

In summary, there are a large number of well-designed trials carried out on adults, but few on young people who are well enough described for clinicians to know to whom they can generalize the findings. This gap in knowledge should be filled. From currently available studies, there is good evidence that antipsychotics can be effective in some children and adolescents, at least to some degree and at least in the short term for the acute management of episodes. Practice parameters for bipolar disorder in young people suggest that both antipsychotics and mood stabilizers may be considered (McClellan et al., 2007). Comparisons between antipsychotics and mood stabilizers favour antipsychotics, but the adverse effect profile makes careful treatment planning needed.

The apparently small effect of lithium and antiepileptics is puzzling in view of the contrast with studies in adults. It may suggest a different basis for mania in young people, or problems in the diagnosis, or an overcautious approach to dosage levels.

Prescribing

Drug treatment should usually begin with an antipsychotic at low dosage (e.g. risperidone, aripiprazole, or quetiapine). In severe cases, and especially when there is psychotic symptomatology, an antipsychotic will be needed for the initial control of symptoms, and can be given orally. There may be a preference for aripiprazole if there are particular risks for metabolic adverse effects, such as obesity or a family history of diabetes.

If the response is not good but the drug was reasonably well tolerated, then consider changing to another antipsychotic. Combination therapy may well be justified. In one study an open trial with a mood stabilizer was followed after 8 weeks by another drug—a second mood stabilizer, a neuroleptic, a stimulant, or an antidepressant according to the remaining pathology (more than half the subjects had ADHD as well). Some 80% were then regarded as showing a good response (Kowatch et al., 2003). In extreme cases, refractory even to combinations of drugs, the use of clozapine can be justified.

If emergency tranquillization is necessary, the choice lies between the a markedly sedative neuroleptic such as olanzapine (which can be given as a rapidly acting tablet dispersible in the mouth), or the combination of risperidone with a sedative benzodiazepine such as lorazepam. The latter combination has the advantage that higher and parenteral doses of lorazepam can be given if required, while olanzapine should not be combined in this way. Intensive monitoring of cardiovascular and respiratory status is required during the hazardous procedure of tranquillization in emergencies.

For longer-term prophylaxis of mania, anticonvulsants and lithium are the best established agents from adult psychiatry, but have little benefit for depression, which is often the most distressing and handicapping aspect of the illness (Yatham et al., 2005). Unfortunately, well-controlled evidence has not appeared to guide clinicians on whether they are effective in young people. Open prospective studies and review of chart records have suggested that a proportion of young people may respond with divalproate (Henry et al., 2003), lithium (Strober et al., 1995), or either lithium or carbamazepine (Dailey et al., 2005). One random-allocation trial found no difference between divalproex sodium and lithium in the outcome for 60 young people aged 5 to 17 with bipolar I or II over a period of 18 months (Findling et al.,

2005). In the absence of an untreated group it is hard to interpret whether this indicates that both are effective or that neither is. In a randomized trial carried out on 40 adolescents who had responded acutely to lithium, Kafantaris et al. (2004) found that placebo-controlled discontinuation was not significantly worse than continued lithium.

The choice of long-term drug is likely to be guided by the adverse event profile of drugs and the individual person's vulnerability to them. In particular, the potential of valproate to cause foetal abnormalities and ovarian problems (McIntyre et al., 2003) suggests that that drug should not be used for girls and women. Quetiapine is well worth considering, especially when its antidepressant properties are desirable for the individual case and when an antipsychotic has been well tolerated and effective in the acute treatment phase (Calabrese et al., 2005). Lurasidone may be an alternative (Loebel et al., 2014).

Psychosocial management should not be neglected. Psychoeducation for the family and the child has several purposes (Fristad, 2006). It can help to alert them to early signs of mania appearing and therefore to prompt treatment. Stress management techniques should help affected people to manage the early stages and possibly to delay relapse. Miklowitz et al. (2003) report the results of a 2-year randomized controlled trial that compared 21 family-based sessions of psychoeducation, communication training, and problem-solving skills training with three sessions of family treatment intended to prevent relapse. Both groups received careful medication. The more intensive treatment gave real benefits in a quicker recovery of depressive symptoms and less time spent in depression. Effects on manic episodes were not significantly different between the groups, but the effects are particularly noteworthy because depression (and accompanying irritability) is often the most disabling part of the disorder.

Chronic, non-episodic states of irritability

Based on the premise that mania may present differently in young people than in adults, some researchers have suggested that chronic non-episodic irritability is a core characteristic of bipolar disorder in young people

In response to the bipolar controversy, Leibenluft et al. (2003) conceptualized chronic irritability as SMD, a category generated to allow for testable comparisons with bipolar disorder. SMD is characterized by chronic and severe irritability with frequent and developmentally inappropriate temper outbursts, along with negatively valenced mood in between outbursts.

Follow-up studies contradicted the notion that severe irritability is an early manifestation of mania. Children with SMD at the age of 10 years suffered from unipolar depression but not bipolar disorder at the age of 18 (Leiben-luft et al., 2006). Stringaris et al. (2009a) reproduced this finding using a 20-year follow-up study. However, these studies were of community samples where the rates of bipolar disorder are low. Therefore, the fact that an association was not found between bipolar disorder and chronic irritability may have been due to the lack of statistical power. To address this, Stringaris et al. (2010a) used a referred sample to compare the course of children with SMD and those with bipolar disorder over a median period of 29 months. The authors found that only one out of 84 (1.2%) of the patients with SMD experienced a manic episode over this time period. By contrast, 58 out of 93 (62.4%) patients with bipolar disorder had a manic episode over the same time period. Again, such findings argue against the notion that chronic irritability is a characteristic of bipolar disorder. It will be informative to follow children with SMD further as they pass through the period of maximum risk for bipolar disorder. Consistent with these findings, SMD and bipolar disorder were found to differ in family history (Brotman et al., 2007), with parents of youngsters with narrow-phenotype bipolar disorder being significantly more likely to be diagnosed with bipolar disorder (14/42, 33.3%) than parents of youngsters with SMD (1/37, 2.7%). Formal diagnostic criteria are set out in Box 10.1. This ad hoc operationalization of chronic irritability—with superimposed angry outbursts and additional symptoms overlapping with ADHD- has been used in several studies and tested against the narrow phenotype of bipolar disorder.

Box 10.1 Research diagnostic criteria for severe mood dysregulation

Inclusion criteria

1 Current age 7–17 years, with onset of the syndrome before age 12.

2 Abnormal mood (specifically, anger or sadness), present at least half of the day most days, and of sufficient severity to be noticeable by people in the child's environment (e.g. parents, teachers, peers).

3 Hyperarousal, defined by at least three of the following: insomnia, agitation, distractibility, racing thoughts or flight of ideas, pressured speech, and intrusiveness.

4 Compared to his or her peers, the child exhibits markedly increased reactivity to negative emotional stimuli that is manifest verbally

Box 10.1 Research diagnostic criteria for severe mood dysregulation (continued)

or behaviourally. For example, the child responds to frustration with extended temper tantrums (inappropriate for age and/or precipitating event), verbal rages, and/or aggression toward people or property. Such events occur, on average, at least three times a week.

5 The symptoms in 2, 3, and 4 are currently present and have been present for at least 12 months without any symptom-free periods exceeding 2 months.

6 The symptoms are severely impairing in at least one setting (home, school, or with peers) and are at least mildly impairing in a second setting.

Exclusion criteria

1 Exhibits any of these cardinal manic symptoms:
  • Elevated or expansive mood
  • Grandiosity or inflated self-esteem
  • Episodically decreased need for sleep

2 The symptoms occur in distinct periods lasting more than 1 day.

3 Meets criteria for schizophrenia, schizoaffective disorder, pervasive developmental disorder, or post-traumatic stress disorder.

4 Meets criteria for substance abuse disorder in the past 3 months.

5 IQ < 70.

6 The symptoms are due to the direct physiological effects of a drug of abuse, or to a general medical or neurological condition.

Brotman et al. (2006) analysed data from the Great Smoky Mountains Study (Costello et al., 1996) where SMD was defined by the CAPA interview. They found that SMD was commoner in boys than girls (77.6% male), with a lifetime prevalence of 3.3% in those 9 to 19 years of age (Brotman et al., 2006). This is in some contrast to the usual finding of approximate gender equality in bipolar disorder I.

In a further study (Stringaris et al. 2010a), the hypothesis was tested that children with SMD would be significantly less likely than those with narrow phenotype bipolar disorder to suffer from (hypo-)manic episodes at follow-up. For this purpose the authors compared 84 children with SMD with 93 children with narrowly defined bipolar disorder. These patients were assessed at baseline and at 6-monthly intervals using the relevant K-SADS modules. It was found that at a median follow-up of 28.7 months, only one of 84 SMD subjects experienced a (hypo-)manic or mixed episode during the study; however, the frequency of such episodes was more than 50 times higher in those with narrowly defined bipolar disorder (58/93, 62.4%). By contrast, those with SMD were indeed at risk for depressive disorders. The authors interpreted their data as suggesting that, over a follow-up period of approximately 2 years, young people with SMD are unlikely to develop (hypo-)manic or mixed episodes.

Other characteristics of SMD are considered further in Chapter 12, together with the closely related condition of DMDD. Taken together, the studies suggest that, contrary to previous assertions, children with chronic irritability are not suffering from DSM-5-type bipolar disorder. SMD and narrow phenotype bipolar disorder appear to differ from each other in their longitudinal course and their familial aggregation. Moreover, the analysis of the Great Smoky Mountains Study suggests that SMD is common in the general population of children and adolescents.

However, several things should be noted when interpreting these findings. Firstly, SMD should not be equated with chronic irritability only. It is important to remember that SMD also contains symptoms that overlap with ADHD. However, this overlap may influence the outcomes of SMD—it is not impossible that some of the associations of SMD are mediated through the hyperarousal elements in its criteria.

Secondly, it should be noted that SMD was created ad hoc and is not an empirically derived construct. As such, its boundaries are drawn arbitrarily and might not reflect a natural category. However, this is true of many if not most psychiatric disorders (Pickles et al., 2003), which are arrived at by consensus of experts and are then subjected to empirical validation.

Thirdly, the studies presented so far should not be taken as offering proof of the lack of association between bipolar disorder and SMD. A community-based longitudinal follow-up (Brotman et al., 2006) did not contain enough cases of bipolar disorder at outcome to estimate the statistical associations with SMD. The clinic study of parental diagnoses (Brotman et al., 2007) could be too small and did not contain sibling controls that might have established whether SMD was part of an extended phenotype of BP just as similar designs have identified a broader phenotype in autism (Rutter, 2000). The clinic follow-up (Stringaris, 2010a) may have been too short and conducted in age groups slightly younger than the age of maximum risk to detect the conversion to bipolar disorder.

The concept of SMD was very influential in the decision of the DSM-5 groups to set up a new diagnosis of DMDD, which is the subject of Chapter 12.

Brief affective episodes

Between the uncommon conditions of bipolar I and II disorders on the one hand and the common states of non-episodic irritability on the other lies a group of cases in which irritability, elation, and grandiosity are present in distinct episodes, but for periods of less than 4 days. They are to be diagnosed as 'bipolar disorders not otherwise specified' (BP-NOS).

A programme of studies—the Course and Outcome of Bipolar Illness in Youth (COBY)—is examining the full range of disorders characterized by mood swings, including those with BP-NOS. The programme began with the identification of 263 children and adolescents at a mean age of 13 years. Approximately 35% showed BP-NOS. Two years later, 25% of them had converted to either bipolar I or II, and they also had poorer outcomes and more rapid changes of mood. At the 4-year follow up 38% of them had converted to bipolar I or II (Birmaher et al., 2009). At this point too, BP-NOS was associated with poorer outcomes than the more classical forms of bipolar disorder.

These findings strongly suggest that short episodes in childhood constitute a substantial risk for the development of the serious mental illness of bipolar disorder. Two outstanding clinical questions are unresolved at the time of writing: how short should such an episode be to be regarded in this way and should they be treated prophylactically?

Clinicians will need to make their judgements on these crucial points on an individual basis. In our practice, for episodically irritable children, we give particular weight to the extent to which the irritability is accompanied by euphoria, grandiosity, and the simultaneous presence of the associated features of mania. We ask careful questions and use diaries to assess the length of episodes and check that they are not entirely accounted for as a natural reaction to major disturbance in the child's environment. We will seldom use the diagnosis for episodes lasting for less than 48 hours.

The relationship between irritability and bipolar disorder in the literature: a summary of the main points and open questions

As the overview presented shows, the controversy on bipolar disorder in children and adolescents is based on very practical concerns about the possibilities of over-diagnosis and over-treatment in this age group. The data from clinic studies are hard to reconcile with those from epidemiological studies, and some unusual definitions of manic episodes as well as circular arguments make it difficult to be confident about the robustness of some of the findings presented. However, some conclusions that are relevant to the aims of this thesis are the following:

- The duration of an episode of altered mood seems to matter. While the difference between 2- or 3-day-long episodes of elated mood and a 4-day hypomanic episode may not be great, the differences between chronic, non-episodic irritability and classical mania are substantial.

- It remains unclear whether the differential predictions of constructs such as SMD are due to chronic irritability or due to the presence of other potential confounding factors—especially the presence of ADHD-type symptoms.

Chapter 11

Irritability in depressive disorders

Recent research has shown that irritability is tightly linked with depression, in keeping with long-held views about the possible common origins of these two clinical presentations. In discussing these links it is important to distinguish between *episodic* and *chronic* irritability: episodic irritability refers to anger and touchiness that is out of keeping with a person's usual presentation, while chronic refers to how the person usually appears and is often also referred to as trait irritability. Boxes 11.1 and 11.2 illustrate how irritability may present in different kinds of emotional disorders.

Irritability and depression in adults

Studies in adults have mainly focused on what we would call episodic irritability.

Interest in the connection between anger/irritability and depression appears to be long-standing; the earliest indication may be found in Burton's work *The anatomy of melancholy*. He saw anger as an important symptom of melancholia:

> facile irascibiles, testy, petty, peevish, and ready to snarl upon every small occasion (Burton, 1932, p. 391)

A particular motivation for a lot of the work on the relationship between depression and irritability in the twentieth century was probably Freud's *Mourning and melancholia* (Freud, 1915). There, Freud proposes that melancholia entails the redirection against the self of aggressive impulses originally directed toward others. In Freud's own words (the original in German with my own translation into English):

> Die unzweifelhaft genußreiche Selbstquälerei des Melancholie bedeutet ... die Befriedigung von sadistischen und Haßtendenzen, die einem Objekt gelten und auf diesem Wege eine Wendung gegen die eigene Person erfahren haben. (Freud, 1915, p. 438)
>
> The undoubtedly pleasurable self-torture of melancholy means the gratification of sadistic and hate tendencies that are directed against an object and, through this way, undergo a transformation to become directed against the self.

Box 11.1 A girl with obsessive–compulsive disorder and irritability

Cindy is an 11-year-old typically developing girl who was doing very well until about a year ago when she started getting worried that she may get infected by germs and that she could pass on the illness to members of her family. She washes her hands up to 50 times a day and uses up a whole bag of liquid soap every day. Her mother describes her as 'the most calm and caring girl you can imagine'; however, in the last 6 months Cindy has become very irritable and shouts at her parents. All of the arguments between Cindy and her parents are about hand washing. Her parents are very concerned because of the damage that Cindy causes to her skin by washing excessively and try to stop her. Cindy feels that something awful will happen if she were to stop washing her hands and she becomes extremely upset. Cindy's symptoms of obsessive–compulsive disorder improved and her irritability was also successfully treated with seven sessions of cognitive behavioural therapy based on exposure and response prevention.

Box 11.2 A girl with depression and irritability

Jane is a 16-year-old girl with a 2-year history of 'feeling low'. She reports feeling low 'all of the time', although she has clearly had at least two episodes where she was particularly depressed and during one of them she came close to being admitted because she had strong suicidal ideation. She often thinks about 'why things are going so wrong' and recalls several incidents, some from the distant past, where people have said negative things about her. She dwells on such events from the past and gets annoyed about the fact that she becomes low or angry. She has severed her relationships with several of her friends who were either involved in such incidents or witnessed her getting 'embarrassingly angry'. She thinks that she is oversensitive, but says that 'the anger and the sadness go hand in hand, when it happens I just can't help it'. Jane's anger improved at the same time as her sadness improved on a combination of fluoxetine and behaviour activation. She found additional sessions focusing on the treatment of angry rumination particularly helpful.

Freud's work itself was based on a previous theory of Karl Abraham, stating that the guilt that is typical of manic–depressive patients resulted from the repression of violent and sadistic impulses (Abraham, 1911). However, empirical studies mainly conducted in the 1970s raised doubts about the validity of this view of anger and hostility turned inwards. In particular, it was found that depressed patients were capable of overt hostility; thus casting doubt on the idea that depressive hostility was directed inwards (Paykel, 1971). Moreover, contrary to psychoanalytic prediction, it was found that, compared with controls, the hostility of depressed patients was indeed directed against those who, in Freudian terms, would be love objects—the patient's spouse or children in particular (Weissman et al., 1971).

More recently, Fava et al. (2010) studied irritability in a large (n = 9282) community-based sample, the National Comorbidity Survey Replication (NCS-R), by comparing the characteristics of patients with depression who had or did not have irritability. Their findings suggest that irritability in the absence of sad mood or anhedonia was rare in the presence of other symptoms of *major depressive disorder (MDD)*. However, compared with those without irritability, subjects with irritable MDD had an earlier (retrospectively ascertained) age at onset of depression and were more likely to show fatigue and symptoms of self-reproach or guilt than those without. Also, irritable MDD was more common than non-irritable MDD among the younger subjects (age range 18–44) and those who had never married. Subjects with irritable MDD also had higher rates of comorbidity overall and with anxiety disorders (most notably generalized anxiety disorder) and impulse control disorders; there was some evidence of higher persistence.

More recently, Judd et al. (2013) compared patients with depression who had irritability with those with depression without irritability using 31-year follow-up data from the National Institute of Mental Health Collaborative Depression Study (n = 536). Close to 55% of patients had irritability at intake. These patients suffered from more severe and more enduring depression, higher comorbidity rates (particularly substance abuse and anxiety), and more antisocial personality disorders. Although patients with depression were more likely to have relatives with bipolar II disorder, the severity of their impairment was independent of any manic symptoms or other comorbidity.

Episodic irritability and depression in children

The research that comes closest to the studies in adults is a study by Stringaris et al. (2013) on episodic irritability in children with depression.

DSM-IV and DSM-5 grant episodic irritability an equal status to low mood as a cardinal criterion for the diagnosis of depression in young people.

This is the only difference between the diagnosis of depression in children and adults. The reason for this difference can be traced back to an old notion that in children depression might present under a different guise—depression could present as enuresis, encopresis, or conduct problems (Malmquist, 1971). While the concept of such 'masked depression' has not stood up to scrutiny, several DSM committees have decided that irritability—instead of sad mood—may be how depression presents in children. However, evidence for irritability as a major criterion of depression in young people is lacking. Stringaris et al. (2013) used data from the prospective population-based Great Smoky Mountains Study (n = 1420). They divided observations on 9–16-year-olds who met criteria for a diagnosis of depression into three groups: those with depressed mood and no irritability, those with irritability and no depressed mood, and those with both depressed and irritable mood. The authors found that depressed mood was the most common cardinal mood in young people meeting criteria for depression (58.7%), followed by the co-occurrence of depressed and irritable mood (35.6%), while irritable mood alone was rare (5.7%). This suggested that very few cases of depression would be missed if irritable mood were no longer considered a cardinal symptom of depression. Boys were more likely to have depressed mood with irritability than were girls. Youngsters with depressed and irritable mood were similar in age and developmental stage to those with depression. This argues against the notion that early onset depression would be more likely to present with irritability rather than sad mood (although the sample did not examine cases that went as far back as early childhood). However, Stringaris et al. (2013) also found that those with depression and irritability had significantly higher rates of disruptive disorders. Nearly 50% of those with depression and irritability had a comorbid ODD or conduct disorder, more than double the rate of these comorbidities in the depressed-only group. So, similarly to what is found in adults, episodic irritability is a common symptom of depression, rarely occurs in the absence of depressed mood, and is linked with increased comorbidity and impairment.

Should irritability be seen as a subtype of depression? So far, distinguishing subtypes in depression has yielded mixed results. The studies quoted did not find evidence of a distinctive symptom profile in those with irritable depression, which argues against irritability being a subtype.

Clinical observation and personal experience suggest that irritability is a mood distinct from depression, although the two have long been known to co-occur in the same individuals. This tight but ambiguous relationship between the two phenotypes is also reflected in the psychological literature about personality: the dimension of negative affectivity refers to a spectrum of aversive emotions that includes both anger (as the distinguishing feature of irritability) and sadness (as the hallmark of depression). Yet another related strand of psychological literature distinguishes between irritability and sadness along a dimension of approach–withdrawal. This distinction resonates with clinical observations about the possible consequences of an irritable state of mind (e.g. fighting with others) as opposed to those of depressed mood (e.g. reduced activity and motivation). It is possible that distinguishing between specific mood states may help to optimize treatment, although there is also evidence that existing treatments may work for both sad as well as irritable mood (Krebs et al., 2013).

Chronic irritability and depression in young people

The interest in the relationship between chronic irritability and depression arises from one of the major puzzles in psychopathology, namely the transition from disruptive behaviour problems to mood and anxiety problems. Strikingly, childhood oppositionality and conduct problems, rather than early depression, are the most robust predictor of young adult depression (Copeland et al., 2009; Stringaris et al., 2014). In 2009, Stringaris and colleagues proposed that irritable mood may explain this transition from oppositionality to later depression (Stringaris et al., 2009b,d). Their data and those of others suggest that oppositionality in young people comprises at least two dimensions with differential predictions: an irritable dimension, more strongly associated with depressive disorders than with antisocial behaviours, and a headstrong/hurtful dimension (capturing argumentativeness and rule breaking alongside spiteful behaviours), more strongly associated with antisocial behaviours than with depressive disorders (see Chapter 9).

The mechanisms underlying this association remain unclear. One possibility is that depression is secondary to irritability. Irritable children may behave in ways that put them at increased risk for depression. They may, for example, be annoying peers, respond angrily to teachers, or get into trouble with the police. This is a so-called failure pathway into depression, where more-or-less self-generated environments play the main role (Capaldi, 1992). Whilst plausible, some findings argue against this model. As we have seen previously, headstrong and hurtful behaviours—which are very plausible candidates for creating such environments—are not significant predictors of depression, once irritability has been accounted for. An alternative—genetic—explanation for the association between depression and irritability has been proposed by Stringaris et al. (2012b). Based on the findings of previous genetic studies concerning the overlap of anxiety and depression, they postulated that so-called 'generalist genes' (Eley, 1997) may underlie the association between depression and irritability. These have been shown to explain the association between other closely linked phenotypes. The authors tested this hypothesis in a twin sample—which allows for the distinction between genetic and environmental influences on the relationship between depression and irritability. They confirmed previous findings demonstrating that irritability showed a significantly stronger phenotypic relationship with depression than with delinquency, whereas headstrong/hurtful behaviours were more strongly related to delinquency than to depression. Moreover, they found that irritability and depression overlapped because they shared genetic effects. Irritability was genetically related to depression significantly more strongly than headstrong/hurtful behaviours were with depression. By contrast, headstrong/hurtful behaviours were genetically much more strongly linked with delinquency than irritability was with delinquency. This study therefore demonstrated that the overlap between depression and irritability is due to shared genetic factors. But it also opened up a number of other questions. First, it is unclear which genes explain the overlap between irritability and depression. It would be important to know which cognitive or other neural mechanisms these genes may code for. Secondly, while genetic effects underlie the link between irritability and depression, environmental effects seem much more important in making irritability distinct from depression. It is unclear what such environments might be.

Indeed, identifying the overlap and differences between irritability and depression promises to be a fascinating area of research. A plausible candidate for the overlap between depression and irritability may be components of the threat network described in Chapter 6. This evolutionarily conserved circuit of areas that include the amygdala, hypothalamus, and periaqueductal grey may function as a generic detector of threat that mobilizes the organism and facilitates cognitive and physical alertness. As we indicated in Chapter 6, whether a response will be one of fear and sadness or one of irritability may largely depend on environmental contingencies. Fear or depression would arise if escape or helpless withdrawal were the only available options, whereas irritability might arise if the outcome prospects of fighting were positive. The probabilities of success, failure, or escape may be calculated as part of a reward valuation processing that occurs in the orbitofrontal cortex.

How would this translate into inter-individual differences. It is plausible to assume that the *appraisal* or *valuation* of environmental contingencies varies between individuals. This may be due to situational effects, but may also be due to more systematic and long-standing experiences. For example, children who have repeatedly experienced the reward of getting their way after having a tantrum or engaging in a punch-up may more readily appraise an ambiguous situation as one where fighting is worthwhile. This would be in keeping with findings about social information bias in models of aggressive behaviour (Dodge et al., 1987).

It is also possible that such biases due to prior experiences are amplified through secondary cognitive processes. Angry rumination may amplify an irritable disposition, whereas sad rumination may bring about yet more sadness and withdrawal.

At a neurotransmitter level, it is important to note that serotonin may be part of the generic arousal process linked to both depression and sadness. Interestingly, serotonin depletion—typically used to induce depression—is at least as potent an inducer of irritability. This links in with treatment studies suggesting that fluoxetine may be a good treatment for at least some forms of irritability (see Treatment).

It should also be noted that while the overlap between depression and irritability is nearly entirely accounted for by genetic effects, irritability and depression each also have genetic effects that are unique to them. Such effects—which may for example manifest in temperamental forms of proneness to aggression—would also shape appraisal and responses following activation of the threat circuit.

Treatment of irritability in depression

There are no data that have looked specifically at the treatment of irritability in depressed children. The clinical impression is that irritability improves as other symptoms of depression do following treatment with serotonin reuptake inhibitors (SRIs) and cognitive behavioural therapy (CBT) or interpersonal therapy (IPT). There is also indirect scientific evidence that SRIs and CBT may be helpful with treating irritability. A Cochrane meta-analysis has found that SRIs are efficacious in treating pre-menstrual dysphoria (Brown et al., 2009), a condition mainly encountered in adult women which is characterized by irritability and mood lability. Also, in a case series Krebs et al. (2013) found that temper outbursts in children with obsessive–compulsive disorder (OCD) were strongly linked with the comorbidity of depression and that both temper outbursts and depression improved with CBT in parallel to the improvement of OCD symptoms. As discussed, the efficacy of modulating serotonin in both depression and irritability is plausible from the perspective of neurobiological theory.

Irritability is important not only as a treatment target in depression, but also as a possible side effect or hindrance to treatment.

Irritability during SRI treatment is often seen as part of an activation that may be associated with the occasionally observed increase in suicidality during treatment. Clinicians will often discontinue SRI treatment out of worry that a young person's irritability may be the harbinger of mania or an indicator of suicidality. It should be stressed that good-quality adult trial data did not find irritability to be associated with an increased liability to a manic switch during treatment (Perlis et al., 2009). So, while the presence of new-onset irritability should always prompt the clinician to exclude the emergence of SRI-induced mania, it should not in and of itself be a reason to stop treatment. Irritability in the absence of elation is relatively rare (Hunt et al., 2009) and should not be labelled as a sign of mania in the absence of other major manic symptoms. When assessing irritability and emergent suicidality one should remember that the number needed to treat depression with SRIs is around 1:10, whereas the number required to induce suicidal ideation (number needed to harm) is close to 1:140 (Maughan et al., 2013). Moreover, this number needed to harm is about suicidal ideation, which is obviously different from suicide attempts, let alone completed suicides. Again, caution and tight suicide monitoring is required when encountering new-onset irritability during treatment, but it is not a good reason in and of itself to deprive patients of a potentially beneficial treatment.

Our own experience has been that irritability often emerges as severely depressed patients who were anergic and apathetic at the onset of treatment improve. It is indeed a sign of activation expressed as annoyance with one's environment (and potentially one's therapist), but it also coincides with the more useful behaviour activation that is so much part of the recovery. We often observe that patients remain dysphoric or anxious (certainly by self-report) while being active, and that this is soon followed by complete recovery. Clearly, the times of maximal dysphoria and increased activity are particularly worrying, but this may be an inevitable risk during recovery. It calls for proactive risk management rather than avoidance. It is also important to note that we have observed this in patients treated exclusively with CBT, so it may not be a direct effect of medication but rather a feature of the recovery. If, however, the irritability persists and therapeutic benefits do not become evident by weeks 3–5 of treatment, then, following recent trial results (Brent et al., 2008), switching to another SRI is indicated. If two SRIs have not worked or worked only minimally, then the clinician should consider extrapolating downwards in age the results from augmentation trials (e.g. with quetiapine, for depression) or other alternative treatments.

Another frequent concern is that the presence of irritability may be a hindrance to the psychological treatment of depression, mainly because it may hinder therapeutic alliance or because frustration may impede CBT homework or behavioural procedures. This has not been systematically studied. However, the work by Krebs et al. (2013) suggests that irritability is not an obstacle to treatment and Chapter 15 also provides meta-analytic evidence in favour of CBT. Indeed, it is possible that the presence of anger becomes a treatment goal in its own right. Novel CBT approaches targeting angry rumination appear to be particularly promising (Leigh et al., 2012) and would be in keeping with theories about the co-occurrence of irritability and depression.

In summary, there is clearly a lot more work that needs to be done to understand and treat irritability in relation to depression. Until such data become available clinicians should proactively treat depression with medication and CBT.

Chapter 12

Irritability and disruptive mood dysregulation disorder

Chronic irritability and frequent temper outbursts with an onset in early childhood are (together with dysphoria) the hallmarks of disruptive mood dysregulation disorder (DMDD). It is one of the new categories in DSM-5 and is classified as a mood disorder.

Background

The main motivation of the American Psychiatric Association (APA) for creating an irritability category originated in the so-called pediatric bipolar debate summarized in Chapter 10. The DSM-IV criteria for mania, requiring a 'distinct period of abnormally and persistently elevated, expansive or irritable mood', were being widely disregarded in practice. There was corresponding concern that many children with chronic irritability were being misdiagnosed as suffering from bipolar disorder. The APA attempted to tackle the dramatic increase of bipolar diagnoses in young people, and the corresponding use of antimanic medication, by introducing DMDD.

The other motivation of the APA for creating DMDD was to provide a diagnostic home for children with severe irritability. These children are deemed to be severely impaired, but their irritability was not codeable under DSM-IV. Irritability, while a presenting problem for many young people (Stringaris, 2011), was either ignored or subsumed under conduct and oppositional disorders. Recognizing irritability as a mood and extreme irritability as a mood disorder is in keeping with a long tradition in psychopathology (Bleuler, 1983) that puts irritability alongside depression and elation as basic moods. It is also in line with psychological research (Stringaris, in press), where anger is one of the basic emotions.

Description of DMDD

The DSM-5 criteria for the new condition of DMDD stress that its core feature is persistent irritability which is both chronic and severe. A child must have had the combination of severe temper outbursts and an enduring mood of anger or irritability even between the temper outbursts for at least 12 months.

The outbursts themselves need to be out of keeping with what is expected for the child's developmental age, and this should be occurring (on average) at least three times a week. The verbal rages or physical aggression must be disproportionate to the situations that provoke them.

The enduring angry mood needs to have been present and observable to others 'most of the day, nearly every day'. There should have been no period as long as 3 months in the year in which the symptoms were absent.

The outbursts and the anger need to be observable in more than one setting (i.e. not only at home or at school or when with peers). The age of onset needs to have been before 10 years, but clinicians are cautioned not to make a diagnosis until the child is 6 years or older. It is a condition of young people and so should not be diagnosed for the first time after the age of 18 years. (This appears to exclude people who present after the age of 18 but with a long history of the problems before that age.) Furthermore, the diagnosis should not be made if the symptoms only occur during an episode of major depressive disorder, or if there has ever been a full day or more during which there were clear manic features or indeed any diagnosis of bipolar disorder, mania, or hypomania. It can, however, co-exist with the presence of major depression, as with ADHD, conduct disorder, and substance misuse.

DSM-5 drew heavily on the formulation of 'severe mood dysregulation' (SMD), which is not an official diagnosis but was created by Leibenluft et al. (2011) as a means of empirically scrutinizing the notion that chronically irritable children may be suffering from bipolar disorder. It is therefore described in Chapter 10. SMD and DMDD overlap considerably, but there are two main differences. One is that in SMD the requirement is for persistent negative mood (Box 10.1, inclusion criterion 2), which may be either irritability or sadness, whereas in DMDD only irritability or anger qualify. The other difference is that DMDD does not include a hyper-arousal criterion (criterion 3 for SMD in Box 10.1). It was omitted in order to reduce confusion with ADHD.

Research findings

Little research has been done on DMDD itself. Most of what we know about severe irritability as a category comes from the research done on SMD (see Chapter 10).

Prevalence

We have discussed the prevalence of the symptom of irritability and of related constructs. The only study so far that estimates the prevalence of a *diagnosis* of DMDD is that by Copeland et al. (2013): using data from two different datasets they found a diagnostic prevalence of between 0.8% and 1.1% for children between 9 and 17 years. These low figures may even be an over-estimate because the authors of the study used a provisional version of the diagnosis, which differed from the final and official one in that it included 'sadness or irritability', rather than chronic irritability only, as the enduring mood criterion for DMDD. However, the authors also show that the prevalence would reach 3.3% if DMDD were diagnosable in preschoolers. Another important finding from this study was that children with DMDD suffered substantial psychosocial impairment and required high levels of service use. Furthermore, DMDD co-occurred with another disorder (mainly depression and ODD) between 60 and 90% of the time and co-occurred with emotional and behavioural disorders in over 65% of cases.

Aetiology

There are no research findings available yet on DMDD as such. However, it is useful to discuss the aetiology of DMDD on the basis of the data available for SMD and dimensional constructs of irritability. We refer readers to other chapters, such as Chapter 6 (neuroscience), Chapter 10 (bipolar disorder), and Chapter 11 (depression), where these questions are discussed in more detail. Here we consider a question that has preoccupied nosologists since the publication of DSM-5, namely, how separable is DMDD from other psychiatric disorders? As we have seen, up to 90% of children with DMDD also have another psychiatric disorder. Some of this association is due simply to item overlap: DMDD has temper outbursts as its main criterion and anger is one of its characteristics, and both these symptoms are also listed as criteria for ODD. Irritability, however, is not only a secondary phenomenon to other disorders. Severe irritability is highly predictive of future impairment and future psychopathology, even after controlling for other disorders (Stringaris et al., 2009b; and see Chapter 5). The distinction from bipolar disorder in symptoms and developmental course has been highlighted in Chapter 10. In keeping with these findings, SMD and bipolar disorder were found to differ in family history. Brotman et al. (2007) compared parental diagnoses in two groups: children with narrow phenotype bipolar disorder and children with SMD. The sample was a referred group of children with either diagnosis, ascertained using the K-SADS interview to establish children's diagnoses and the Diagnostic Interview for Genetic Studies to establish parental diagnoses. The clinicians interviewing the parents were blind to the diagnoses of the offspring. Thirty-three children with bipolar disorder and 42 parents were compared with 30 children with SMD and 37 parents. The authors found that compared with parents of children with SMD, parents of youngsters with narrow phenotype bipolar disorder were significantly more likely to be diagnosed with bipolar disorder. In particular, 14 out of 42 (33.3%) parents of children with narrow phenotype bipolar disorder had a lifetime diagnosis of bipolar disorder; however, only 1 out of 37 (2.7%) parents of children with SMD were found to be suffering from bipolar disorder. The difference was statistically significant with an odds ratio of 17.96 (CI 1.89–170.77). They did not find any other differences between the two groups.

Brotman et al. (2007) note some of the study's limitations, such as its small sample size and the lack of an unaffected control group. They conclude that the narrow phenotype bipolar disorder may be distinct from SMD in terms of familial aggregation.

Regarding the genetics and neuroscience of irritability, we refer readers to Chapter 4 and 5, respectively.

Management and differential diagnosis

For management please refer to Chapter 3 on the assessment of irritability. There is as yet no specific instrument to measure DMDD. Differential diagnosis is discussed in Chapter 14.

Treatment

There is as yet no licensed treatment for DMDD and the evidence base for treating severe irritability is thin.

As with most medical conditions, it is important that the clinician provides adequate information about the condition, its likely causes, and treatment. This is best done in the form of psychoeducation, where the clinician cooperates with the patient and the carers to achieve optimal communication and information sharing. While psychoeducation has yet to be tested as an intervention in DMDD, it is part of effective treatments for other conditions (Miklowitz et al., 2008) and has also been shown to be effective in adult samples with other disorders (Colom et al., 2003). Its benefits are partly derived through better adherence to treatment.

Identifying conditions that may underlie severe irritability or contribute to it (as discussed) is an important first step in the treatment of children with severe irritability. A recent study suggests that severe tantrums in children with OCD respond to standard treatment with CBT (Krebs et al., 2013).

Similarly, it appears that irritability and mood fluctuations in some children with ADHD may respond to treatment with stimulants (Blader et al., 2009).

However, many children with DMDD will not improve with treatment of any comorbid condition. An adequately powered study has concluded that lithium is not effective in children with SMD (Dickstein et al., 2009). The role of selective SRIs in treating severe irritability in young people is unclear and the results of an ongoing trial at the NIH are awaited (Dr Ellen Leibenluft, NIMH, personal communication). Sodium valproate appears effective in young people with ADHD whose aggression has not responded to stimulant treatment (Blader et al., 2009), although its effectiveness in irritability has yet to be demonstrated. Antipsychotic medications, such as risperidone and aripiprazole, have been used successfully to treat irritability in people with ASD (McCracken et al., 2002) and learning difficulties; however, it is not clear how much the irritability construct in these studies overlaps with irritability in typically developing children. An open-label trial using low doses (1.2 ± 0.5 mg) of risperidone in children and adolescents with SMD showed significant reductions in irritability scores (Krieger et al., 2011), yet any benefits of such treatment should be balanced against its downsides, such as sedation and metabolic complications.

Parenting interventions (e.g. based on Webster-Stratton techniques) have been shown to be effective in children with ODD (Pilling et al., 2013). It also seems that children who suffer from ODD and show predominantly irritability may benefit specifically from parenting interventions (Scott et al., 2012), although this needs to be tested further.

Treating anger with CBT seems moderately effective according to meta-analytic studies (Lochman et al., 2011). In our experience using a functional analysis of behaviour to identify circumstances during which tantrums occur can be very helpful; similarly, characterizing the cognitions (particularly ruminative thoughts) that accompany anger and persistent irritability appears helpful in reducing symptoms of anger (Leigh et al., 2012), although the effectiveness of these approaches has yet to be formally tested in children with DMDD. Clinicians treating children with DMDD will want to address treatable comorbidities. We refer the reader to the chapters on other conditions such as ADHD in which irritability frequently occurs. An overview of specific treatments for irritability is given in Chapter 14.

Chapter 13

Irritability in brain disorders and brain damage

Acquired brain injury

Unprovoked outbursts of aggression are very common as one part of the behavioural changes that follow injury to the brain. In the early stages of recovery, often in hospital, they accompany disorientation and confusion. In the later stages of recovery they can be very disruptive of rehabilitation. The literature on adults makes it plain that aggressive outbursts can persist for long periods after injury. Tateno et al. (2003) found that a third of their patients had significant problems of aggression during the first 6 months after injury. This was three times the rate for those with multiple injuries that spared the brain. Baguley et al. (2006) found that a quarter of their head-injured patients were still having similar problems at the 5-year follow-up.

Not all aggression, of course, is driven by anger. A distinction has often been made between instrumental and hostile aggression, the latter type being explosive, agitated, and with little provocation or manipulative effect (see the critique by Bushman and Anderson, 2001). It is this 'hostile' type that is most characteristic of the effects of a brain injury (Silver et al., 2011) and closest to the theme of this book.

Similar problems in children have received rather little scientific study. Clinical experience suggests that for them, as well as adults, acquired brain injury has both immediate consequences in confusional states and long-term consequences in personality changes (Max et al., 1997), and both kinds of sequelae include irritability and hostile aggression. Importantly, the later sequelae in mental health seem to be predicted not only by the severity of the injury but also by some aspects of family reaction (Lax Pericall et al., 2014). Parents may be profoundly sad at the loss of the way their child used to be, may be blaming themselves for the cause of the head injury, and may find it hard to restrain a tendency to overprotect their child thereafter or to maintain firmness in discipline. Others may press urgently for the restoration of the previous function of the child, with the unintended result of creating frustration and poor self-esteem. Most, of course, offer the injured child the best of the support that comes from any source.

The nature of the psychiatric problem does not follow closely on the localization of the injury. A follow-up of penetrating head injuries in children found little relationship between site and psychiatric presentation (Shaffer et al., 1975), apart from a possible over-representation of depression in those with right frontal lesions. The severity of the lesion was a more important influence. This study, admittedly, was done before the availability of magnetic resonance imaging that might have found a clearer relationship. Nevertheless, the effect of injury is seldom confined to a single part of the brain. *Contre-coup* effects (resulting from the to-and-fro motion of the shocked brain) and shearing effects stemming from rotational forces will often make for diffuse brain lesions.

Management of the explosive states of anger and agitation in children will follow the general rules of Chapter 14, but with some specific considerations. Psychological management will usually focus on family support—which should be respectful and individually designed—and advice to educators, often involving information about the cognitive effects of injury that may well be present too.

Pharmacological management has some evidence base from studies of adults. Fleminger et al. (2006) provide a Cochrane Review of drugs for agitation and aggression in acquired brain injury. Most of the randomized controlled trials available to them were comparing a beta-blocker (such as propranolol) with a placebo, and there were beneficial effects of the active drug. There was some evidence of benefit for carbamazepine, and lamotrigine is also sometimes used. Indeed, these anticonvulsants seem to be used much more widely than the beta-blockers, which have the advantage of more evidence and fewer adverse effects. Sedation from anticonvulsants, or even more from neuroleptics, is a particular concern where cognition is already blunted by compromised brain function. Evidence does not tell us whether the same rules apply in childhood and adolescence, but our clinical experience is moderately positive.

Chronic brain syndromes

Challenging behaviour

Irritability is a key part of 'challenging behaviour' (CB). CB is not recognized as such in the main diagnostic schemes, so does not have a standard definition. Nevertheless, CB is widely used as a useful construct by professionals trying to help people with intellectual disability, ASD, epilepsy, and other brain syndromes. As well as severe temper tantrums, the main features are profound non-compliance, self-injurious behaviour, aggression against others, and destruction of property (often in the course of a rage). This pattern is rather distinctive, and it is not identical with that of conduct disorder. People with CB are not usually spiteful (though their aggression may well be misperceived as such by the victims) and antisocial behaviours such as stealing and lying are not usually present.

People with ASD are prone to develop CB, but CB also occurs in many intellectually disabled people who do not have autistic features. In a survey of behaviour problems in children with intellectual disability, irritability was distinct from autistic symptoms, and did not (unlike many other problems) correlate with a lower level of adaptive function (Chadwick et al., 2000). McClintock et al. (2003) reported a meta-analysis of studies describing the risk markers for CB in people with intellectual disabilities. Significant associations included low adaptive function and impaired communication, autistic features, and pain from physical conditions. These need to be considered in the assessment of very irritable children; and they give some clues about the developmental processes involved.

Toothache, earache, stomach pains, and headache are the commonest of the physical triggers, and there should be an examination for them, especially when CB has appeared or worsened acutely. Children with impaired communication skills may well not have indicated their distress in the usual ways.

Communication difficulties can also be a great source of frustration, and a tantrum may be the only ready way of signalling a need. Alternative systems of communication—including sign language and picture boards—are then key tools for education and family life. Environmental changes can be hard to understand or cope with for people with chronic brain syndromes. Even small changes should be recognized as potentially disruptive, explained carefully, and made as gradual as possible.

The psychosocial associations of conduct disorder are conspicuous by their absence in CB. Poverty, large family size, and other antisocial family relatives do not seem to be linked. Even discordant family relationships, if present, usually seem to be consequences of rather than a cause of the disruptive mood states.

The usual methods of parent training, as applied for conduct and oppositional problems and ADHD, are usually ineffective for CB. Insistence on applying them is likely to evoke only a feeling in parents that their problems are not understood. More intensive intervention is needed, directed at analysing the individual problems of the child. Applied behaviour analysis (ABA) requires a specially trained professional to apply the principles of social learning theory (Howlin et al., 2009). Specialized educational units can be an effective way of using individualized behavioural regimes.

Risperidone has been used in several trials in children with subaverage intelligence and disruptive behaviour: it is efficacious in reducing the behaviour problems (Aman et al., 2002, Snyder et al., 2002). Pharmacological treatments for CB have not yet been trialled for the specific circumstance of irritability, but many of the subjects, in trials of drugs in intellectual disability, would probably have met this description. Risperidone and aripiprazole are probably the most efficacious for periods of up to a few months. Long-term medication poses difficult decisions for the prescriber in balancing the benefits against the risks.

Epilepsy

Epilepsy is associated with ADHD, autism, oppositional, conduct, and affective disorders, and any or all of these may need managing when severe tempers are the presentation. In addition, there are considerations specific to the seizures or their treatment.

Emotional seizures

The aura of a seizure may include an emotion of dread or rage. Either can result in a passionate outburst. The site is often, but not exclusively, in the temporal lobes. The key to diagnosis is usually the report of the subjective sensation, which may be accompanied by distortions of perception, abnormal smells, or sensations of unreality. Electroencephalography (EEG) may show abnormalities only during an attack, or not at all. Non-specific EEG 'abnormalities' are common in people who do not have epilepsy. A normal EEG does not exclude, and an abnormal one does not establish, that the abnormal experience is the result of an epileptic seizure.

Automatisms

Automatisms, during or just after a seizure, can include violent aggression. The key to the diagnosis is usually the observation of one such attack by somebody who is either knowledgeable about epilepsy or can give a careful account. Typically, the person is out of touch with the environment during the episode, and the movements are disorganized and unfocused and may be repetitive. They are often followed by a period of confusion. Any speech during the episode is unlikely to make sense, and memory for it is absent or reduced. It can be helpful for an observer to say a distinctive word (e.g. a place name) and see if it can be recalled afterwards.

Auras of anger and ictal aggression are both rare events. Aggression during a psychomotor automatism is usually the result of attempts by others to impose physical restraint (Rodin, 1973). An epileptic origin is much more commonly suspected than found. Routine use of the EEG in people who lack the specific features described is likely to yield only confusion and expense.

Interictal rages—those occurring in a person with epilepsy, but not during a seizure—have a variety of causes, essentially similar to those affecting people without epilepsy. In one series of 44 adult patients with epilepsy, interictal violence was related to co-existent psychopathology and intellectual disability; not to any features of the epilepsy itself (Mendez et al., 1993). Mental health problems, associated with poor anger control, such as ADHD, often precede the onset of seizures (Hesdorffer et al., 2004). There may be long-term influences of seizures themselves upon mental function, for instance in the association between continuous epileptic EEG discharges in sleep and behavioural problems in waking life. A specific impact of seizure frequency or 'kindling' on the frequency of anger outbursts has not yet been found—or indeed examined. The likely reason for the association of epilepsy with severe mental health problems is that both are consequences of underlying brain disorder or damage.

Anticonvulsant drug effects

Effective control of seizures by anticonvulsant medication will sometimes reduce mental health problems—including those related to impaired impulse control. To set against this are the known adverse effects of medication—prominent among which are irritability, sedation, and aggression. These adverse effects are linked to some anticonvulsants more than others. Domizio et al. (1993) reported them in 76% of those treated with phenobarbitone in comparison with 31% of those given different drugs. Drug toxicity can be suspected, especially when blood levels are high, folate levels are low, and several anticonvulsants are being given together.

Interactions between anticonvulsants and psychotropic drugs may also be reducing the effectiveness of the latter. The interactions are drug-specific, and it is very desirable if one prescriber can be responsible for all the medications that are given to modify seizure frequency and mental health status. Good monitoring, and recording over time, can help a prescriber to learn from the effects of changes in the past.

Specific neurological syndromes

Tourette syndrome

This is a neurodevelopmental condition characterized by multiple motor and vocal tics. Brief and angry outbursts are common, and the clinician needs to determine whether they represent complex and involuntary actions, are the result of associated neurodevelopmental disorders (such as ADHD and OCD), or are the same mixtures of genetic and environmental influences that are found in people with normally developing brains. Drug treatments for the tics are typically based on blockade of dopamine or alpha-2 adrenergic transmission—clonidine, risperidone, aripiprazole, haloperidol, and pimozide are all in common use. They can all be expected to have effects in reducing irritability, as described in Chapters 8 and 14. Irritability may therefore be an indication for drug treatment even if the young people are not troubled by the motor and vocal tics themselves.

Anger control techniques (see Chapter 14) are also applicable. A randomized trial, allocating 26 adolescents to receiving either 10 sessions of CBT-oriented approaches (with some optional extra sessions) or to treatment as usual was reported by Sukhodolsky et al. (2009). Disruptive behaviour problems were reduced by some 52% in those receiving anger control measures but only by 11% in those receiving the usual treatment. The improvement was maintained at a 3-month follow-up.

Pseudobulbar palsy

Pseudobulbar palsy is a condition with many causes that impact on motor nuclei in the brainstem and their critical connections. As well as speech problems, difficulty in swallowing, and problems in tongue (and other) movements, affected children often show a high degree of emotional lability. They react excessively and over-frequently with laughter and crying, and may show angry outbursts. Treatments include selective SRIs and dextromethorphan (an NMDA receptor antagonist which inhibits glutamatergic transmission) in combination with quinidine (Brooks et al., 2004).

Smith–Magenis syndrome

This is due to an abnormality of chromosome 17, and includes among its features an abnormal sleep pattern and frequent temper tantrums. The two may be related. Tempers appear to occur particularly during onset of sleep and waking—both of which sleep transitions occur many times a day because of abnormal rhythms of melatonin secretion. Treatment is often with melatonin supplements at night, and suppression of melatonin production in the daytime (e.g. with acebutolol).

Dementias

Irritability can also occur as one feature of the personality changes that result from a variety of progressive neurological diseases, including some that may be treatable: subcortical dementia in HIV, structural lesions such as frontal tumours, systemic lupus erythematosus, Wilson's disease, and metachromatic leucodystrophy. Even for diseases for which treatment is at present only symptomatic (such as Sanfilippo syndrome), early diagnosis can enhance the quality of life for patients and their families.

Chapter 14

Clinical management of irritability and disruptive mood

In Chapter 3 we described the process of obtaining useful information about the mood states and behavioural problems that are presented by irritable children. Clinicians will then wish to move to making a diagnostic formulation—both of the type of mood change present and about the presence or absence of any other types of psychopathology that may be associated. In making a treatment plan they will want to consider the strengths and weaknesses that will determine how far to focus management on the individual child (with psychological treatment or medication) and how far on their social context. The initial stage of clinical contact will end with the formulation of a therapeutic plan, conveying this in suitable terms to the child and the responsible adults, and setting up systems for the monitoring of response to intervention.

Current diagnostic approaches

Angry mood states become considered as abnormal if they are excessive in intensity, frequency, or both, out of keeping with any provocation or with the developmental age of the child, and causing harm to the child or other people. In diagnostic terms, they may be a disorder in themselves, a criterion for a broader diagnosis, or a non-specific accompaniment of a physical or mental disorder (Table 14.1). In the DSM-5 they enter into the diagnosis of several different conditions and this can lead to some confusion about clinical cases in which irritability is a central feature. Scientific work has not yet established secure and validated criteria for the boundaries between them, and will no doubt do so in time. Meanwhile we propose a way of distinguishing them in terms of length of angry episodes, mood between episodes, and the presence of coexisting disorders.

The definitions of *bipolar disorder* have long included irritability—as well as euphoria and grandiosity—as cardinal features of a manic episode. The

Table 14.1 Diagnostic status of conditions of irritability

Irritability as a diagnosis	Intermittent explosive disorder
	Pathological rage
	Severe emotional dysregulation (chronic irritability)
	Disruptive mood dysregulation disorder (chronic irritability)
Irritability as one of several criteria for a disorder	Oppositional–defiant disorder (chronic irritability)
	Mania and hypomania (episodic irritability)
	Depression (episodic irritability)
	Post-traumatic stress disorder
Irritability as a non-diagnostic accompaniment of a psychiatric disorder	ASD
	ADHD
Irritability as a consequence of organic conditions	Epilepsy
	Brain injury and disease
	Confusional states
	Pain
	Sedation

ASD, autism spectrum disorders; ADHD, attention deficit/hyperactivity disorder.

disorder is conceived as episodic, so irritability must have appeared (or worsened) at the same time as the other emotional and behavioural features of mania. There is as yet no clear clinical consensus about what the minimum length of an episode should be to qualify. This question is considered in detail in Chapter 10. For the present purposes we recommend that the irritability should represent clear breaks from normal functioning, should occur in episodes some of which at least should last for 48 hours or more, and should be accompanied by other manic features.

DMDD is described in Chapter 12 and should be considered if the angry outbursts do not include manic features such as euphoria and grandiosity, or are too short for even our relaxed criteria, and are accompanied by an enduring mood change that is resentful, sullen, bad-tempered, or otherwise angry. The new term provides a category to describe *severe* and chronic irritability without the bipolar features of grandiosity, euphoria, and prolonged mood swings.

MDD is described in Chapter 11. The characteristic mood is sad, wretched, or hopeless. There should be caution in diagnosing it if the only mood change is anger.

ODD includes not only the affective features of excessive anger and spitefulness in its definition, but also the behavioural features of defiance and non-compliance. These components are aggregated in the diagnostic criteria, so it is possible to achieve the diagnosis without irritability, or without defiance. Bipolar disorder and DMDD should both be treated as excluding ODD: in effect they include more severe versions of the ODD problems.

Coexisting neurodevelopmental disorders should always be assessed. ADHD, ASD, Tourette syndrome, and learning disabilities can exist alongside bipolar, disruptive mood, and depressive disorders. They can, however, also be causes of severe irritability, so they may become the primary diagnosis if none of the list of bipolar, disruptive mood, and depressive disorders is present. Similarly, physical illnesses (especially those causing pain), substance misuse, and maltreatment should be considered for their contribution to irritability. If these other conditions are sufficient explanations for the angry presentation, then there is of course no need for further diagnostic formulation.

Intermittent explosive disorder (IED) comes at the bottom of the hierarchy of diagnoses. Its essence is that its angry outbursts are not accompanied by any abnormality of mood between times. Since the only evidence for the disorder is the outbursts, it can scarcely be used to explain them or be said to cause them. In practice the term has been used by adult psychiatrists, not by child or adolescent specialists. The current state of development of DSM-5, however, does make IED into a childhood diagnosis by removing any age restrictions on its use. It should not be diagnosed if other conditions are present.

'Pathological rage' has similar connotations to IED; the term has tended to be used to describe provoked but extreme anger (e.g. 'road rage') and to emphasize the extreme nature of the mental state. The phenomenology of rage includes an altered sense of the passage of time ('events in slow motion'), abnormalities of sensation (diminution of pain, and perceptions of enhanced or muffled hearing), and sometimes forgetfulness of what has been done during the episode. The similarity of these to some ictal phenomena has led to the term carrying some implications of neurological origin and being used by neurologists more than by psychiatrists; but no evidence distinguishes it from common-or-garden anger except its severity.

Clinicians therefore have several possible diagnoses for children presenting with abnormal levels of anger that are disproportionate to their context. A flow chart for conditions characterised by excessive episodes of anger is proposed in Fig. 14.1. It suggests beginning by establishing the length of episodes of anger, going on to the mood between outbursts, and then to the presence of other psychological or physical medical conditions. When one of the diagnoses listed is present, then the specific aspects of management are described in the relevant chapters. However, some aspects of management can be considered whether there is an underlying psychiatric diagnosis or not.

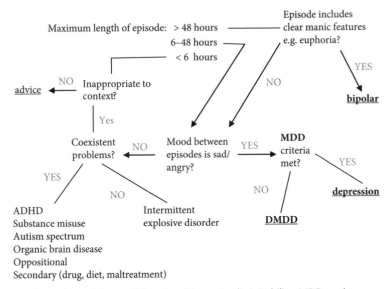

Fig. 14.1 Diagnosis in conditions involving episodic irritability: MDD, major depressive disorder; ADHD, attention deficit/hyperactivity disorder; DMDD, disruptive mood dysregulation disorder.

Psychological and social management

Psychological aspects of management can include the removal or reduction of provoking factors, the modification of the child's response to them, and intervention at the level of prolonged abnormal mood states that may occur even between angry outbursts.

The nature of provoking factors should be borne in mind throughout the assessment. There may be hints from the start in the child's and family's attitudes to referral and to the problems themselves. Attention should be paid not only to what parents are saying about a child but also the manner in which they are saying it. A hostile and critical attitude toward the child is likely to be a factor in encouraging not only angry feelings but also overt aggression. There may be evidence of this from the observation of how families interact or from the ways in which the parents talk about the child in his or her absence. The measurement of expressed emotion by parents has been developed as a reliable research tool requiring specialized training, and some features can be brought into clinical practice. The diagnostic interview can include noting the balance of positive and negative remarks and the emotional tone in which remarks are made. Questions such as 'How have you felt about this problem?' may uncover high levels of criticism; questions such as 'What are the things that you value about him most?' may uncover a lack of warmth in the relationship. Care should be taken to avoid extraneous aspects such as a parent's personability and general social warmth. Expressed criticism/hostility or lack of warmth are intended to be a proxy indication for a negative emotional atmosphere at home. Table 14.2 illustrates how to assess warmth and criticism.

There may also be evidence from the description of what actually happened during recent incidents of rages that will give clues to the antecedents and consequences of the tempers of which the parents are complaining. Questions along the lines of 'And what did you think when he did that?', 'What happened then?', 'What did you do?', or 'How did he/she respond to what you did?', may give information about the sensitivity and the planfulness of parental responses. Such questioning may also uncover considerations such as conscious or unconscious encouragement of the behaviours constituting an angry outburst. Children identified as vulnerable may not be disciplined for fear of harming them or aggressive children may not be disciplined for fear of encouraging further violence. It is important for the clinician to convey an understanding and non-condemnatory attitude during the initial stages of assessment. At this stage, families need to feel that their concerns are being taken seriously and that the position of everyone is being taken into account.

Table 14.2 Warmth and criticism indicators during parental interview

Indicators of warmth	Tone of voice is important. Be alert to: • Enthusiasm shown when talking about the child • A tendency for the parent to stress the child's positive points • A sympathetic, interested concern in the child's problems • An interest in the child's person, and expression of enjoyment of his/her company
Indicators of criticism	Criticism can be rated independently of warmth. Look for: • The parent complains a lot about problems and never mentions the child's good qualities • When mentioning good qualities, the parent frequently adds counterbalancing criticism • The parent criticizes the child's personality rather than behaviour • The parent makes clear rejecting remarks: 'I can't forgive her for doing that', 'I hate him in that mood'

NB: criticism is not inferred simply because problems are repeatedly described, especially if there are unsolicited positive remarks when talking about difficult behaviour (e.g. 'He is disruptive, but he can also be thoughtful').

Data from E. Heptinstall (1991): Manual for the PACS interview. London: Institute of Psychiatry.

The next step may be one of giving basic advice on handling (see Box 14.1). This advice is more effective if done as part of a formal 'parent training' programme. Such programmes are quite widely available in modern health, educational, and social systems; so the family may already have enjoyed such an experience before clinical referral. Where such a programme is not available it may be helpful to indicate and discuss the nature of a rage. A child is not receptive in a rage and there is little point in reasoning or in applying complex behavioural schedules at that point. Rather, a phase of regret, remorse, and guilt quite often follows an extreme temper and at that point—and when the reactions of adults have also calmed—a constructive conversation may be able to be held. At that point, the conversation can be understanding about the angry feelings, suggesting alternative ways of dealing with them, and applying any consequences for the behaviour that had previously been agreed without concentrating on loss of long-term treats for the child or accusations of moral failure.

'Time out' procedures are often recommended in the control of displays of anger. Time, that is, in which the child is removed from rewards that might maintain the behaviour, for example by going to a quiet place without agreeable activities. This can, however, be counterproductive. 'Go to your room' may indeed help as a calming device, but it may also be a reward by removing the child from an unhappy situation. The usual expectation is that when time out procedures are started for aggressive behaviours the frequency of those behaviours will temporarily increase before they decline. Indeed, this may happen to a point where it is intolerable for the family and extreme reactions can follow. Behaviour therapists often recommend a process of rewarding incompatible behaviours in this situation rather than attempting extinction by removing the reward. Simple and well-meant pieces of advice may, if they do not work, create a disillusion in a family that militates against formal psychological help.

Parent training programmes are increasingly well developed and increasingly available. The programmes have several purposes and are intended for several different kinds of problem situations. They do in general seek to promote a warm family atmosphere, collaborative play between parent and child, open communication, and clear and consistent styles of discipline based on the application of achievable rules. Different children probably respond best to different techniques. Aggressive children probably need a system based on firm control and supervision, by contrast with the gentler control that can be appropriate for more anxious children (Kochanska, 1997). Irritable children also seem to respond better to a firmly controlling atmosphere (Bates et al., 1998). Parenting interventions (e.g. based on Webster-Stratton techniques) have been shown to be effective in children with ODD (Pilling et al., 2013). It also seems that children who suffer from ODD and predominantly show

Box 14.1 Handling a childish tantrum

1 *Early recognition*. Younger children will need parents to be aware of building tension; in later childhood and adolescence they should be learning how to recognize it in themselves. There may be only a few seconds in which there is the chance to promote cooling down before a full-blown rage ensues.

2 *Distraction*. An alternative activity needs to be pleasant and attractive. Going straight to something quiet and calm may be too difficult a transition; energetic activity outside followed by a gradual calming may be more realistic.

3 *Offering alternatives, applying consequences*. A plan should have been agreed beforehand. It might involve the child showing a red card to indicate that they need to be left alone, or going to punch cushions, or moving to a favoured activity. Contingencies should also have been negotiated beforehand. If the alternative has been followed, the child is praised and rewarded for having followed the rule. If alternatives have been ignored and a rage has developed, then negative consequences (preferably short-term, e.g. a brief loss of computer game time) should be announced immediately and in an emotionally neutral manner.

4 *Ensuring safety*. A severe and persisting rage may need parents to learn, or apply, safe restraining to prevent injury. If this does become necessary, then as far as possible the parental emotional reaction should not be visible to the child, for example the child should be held from behind.

5 *Applying agreed contingencies after the tantrum ends*—in order to reduce the likelihood of future tantrums rather than end the current tantrum. Response cost is often applied as a removal of points (or stickers, or stars, or counters) in a token economy. 'Over-correction' may be applied as a restitution to people who have been hurt or distressed. These negative consequences should not be excessive or punitive.

6 *Later discussion*. As indicated, when calm is restored there may indeed be the opportunity to develop understanding of the communicative function of the temper, or the situation that led to it. Was the child feeling humiliated or unfairly treated? It may be possible for them to develop a better way of conveying the feeling, or to get a better understanding of the situation, or to work out a way of avoiding it in the future.

irritability may benefit particularly well from parenting interventions (Scott et al., 2012), although this needs to be tested further.

Randomized controlled trials have in general focused on conduct problems broadly defined rather than specifically on irritability. Pilling et al. (2013) have produced a systematic review and meta-analysis of some 54 trials on conduct problems in children of normal intelligence, and concluded that there is indeed a moderate effect size (around 0.5) on antisocial outcomes—at least when rated by parents, who do of course have a vested interest in a positive outcome of the work in which they have been closely involved. It was also concluded that the effect diminished considerably (about half) 1 year after the initial outcome. Furthermore, ratings by teachers showed smaller effects of the parent programmes. Further still, it has been hard to show that the effects of such programmes in the real world, when delivered routinely by generic professionals, have anything like as good an outcome as is achieved in formal trials.

Comparisons of the approaches based on social learning theory with counselling and humanistic processes favour the former (Bank et al., 1991). Directive approaches appear to work better than non-directive ones (Charach et al., 2013).

In summary, we recommend from the evidence base that, after assessment, the parents of irritable children should be referred for parenting programmes (such as Incredible Years or Triple P) that are based on the principles of social learning and on the development of a warm atmosphere, good communication, and consistent discipline. We also note that the evidence base is not strong enough to be able to recommend that this is a sufficient provision by mental health services—many cases will be sufficiently severe that disorder-specific management should start right away.

Approaches directed not to families but to the children themselves focus especially on cognitive behavioural approaches to anger control and the modification of aggressive or violent attitudes. Techniques for anger control are described in detail in several manuals (e.g. Feindler et al., 1986; Deffenbacher et al., 2000). They will typically involve education about recognizing anger triggers and the early signs of developing anger. Once identified, the next step will often be to practise ways of managing the arousal—such as deep breathing, muscle relaxation, and positive imagery. Discussion and exercises contribute to cognitive restructuring of hostile attributions ('Could there have been another reason for that happening?'). Ways of solving the problems that arise for the individual can be worked out ('What other things might be done when people have been disciplined?', 'Could you do anything like that next time?'). Role-playing of situations that have provoked tempers in the past can lead to practise there and then of how to resolve conflict—methods that can then be taken into the real world, practised, and the results written down.

In the evidence base there are reports about the efficacy of individual programmes, such as the SCARE programme reported by Herrmann et al. (2003). A meta-analysis by Sukhodolsky et al. (2004) was based on 21 published and 19 unpublished reports. The mean effect size (0.67) was in the medium range and good enough to bring into clinical practice. Skills training, problem solving, and affective education all had at least moderately good effects, but problem-solving treatments were more effective than the others in reducing subjective experiences of anger.

Pharmacological management of irritability

It is plain that psychological approaches have merit and should be available but that they are not universally or uniformly effective. This, together with the lack of trained therapists, has contributed to the widespread use of medication for children and young people.

When medication is directed specifically at an underlying disorder then it can be very effective, and the results are reviewed in the chapters on specific psychological problems. In the context of this chapter, however, it is necessary to consider the generic use of medication where there is no specific indication other than the presence of irritability and disruptive mood. For this purpose there is a very limited evidence base. We summarize the current state of the evidence in the flow diagram in Fig. 14.2.

Antiepileptics

Antiepileptics are also used as mood stabilizers. Divalproex, other valproate preparations, carbamazepine, and lamotrigine are those best evaluated for this purpose in adults. Serum level estimates are widely available and the dosage should be titrated accordingly: the therapeutic range for valproate is around 80–120 mg/ml. If dosage is not governed by blood tests then the dose for valproate would be 10–20 mg/kg/day in divided doses and for carbamazepine 5 mg/kg/day in divided doses.

Donovan et al. (2000) reported a small trial of divalproex against placebo in 20 subjects aged 10–18 years who combined an oppositional–defiant or conduct disorder with 'explosive' tempers and labile mood. Those assigned to divalproex were more likely to respond well than were those on placebo. Otherwise, there is little in the way of an evidence base for irritable children who do not have bipolar disorder or ASD.

The adverse effects of antiepileptic drugs are possibly less troublesome in the long run than those of the second-generation antipsychotics to be

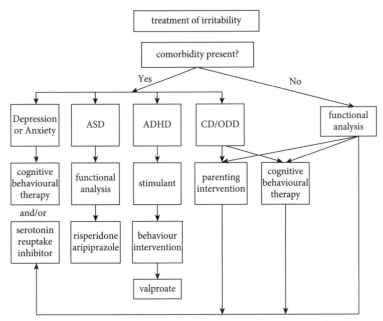

Fig. 14.2 Treatment algorithm for irritability: ASD, autism spectrum disorders; ADHD, attention deficit/hyperactivity disorder; CD/ODD, conduct disorder/oppositional–defiant disorder; CBT, cognitive behavioural therapy; SRI, serotonin re-uptake inhibitor;

described—but are still considerable. Sedation and headache are common events and weight gain is sometimes seen. In females, the dangers of valproate for a foetus or for ovarian function are so great that this particular drug should only be given for otherwise refractory epilepsy, not for the psychiatric complications. Self-harm has been widely publicized as a possible hazard. In a meta-analysis conducted by the FDA (2008) of 11 different antiepileptic drugs used in children and adults for a variety of indications (epilepsy, bipolar disorder, migraine, etc.), the estimated overall odds ratio for suicidal behaviour or ideation among drug-treated versus placebo-treated patients was 1.80 (95% confidence interval 1.24–2.66). (When antiepileptics have been used for the treatment of manic states involving irritability, they have been less effective than low-dose neuroleptics, as described in Chapter 10.)

Antipsychotics

Antipsychotics have a clear place in the treatment of bipolar disorder. They are also widely used, at low doses, for a variety of conditions where the control of agitation, anxiety, and aggression is desired. All the antipsychotics have pharmacological actions in blocking dopamine receptors, and most also act on the serotonin (5HT) receptors. They differ in the details of which dopamine receptors, and which others, receive the blockade (see Table 14.3). There is trial evidence for efficacy in severe irritability in ASD (see Chapter 8) and/or intellectual disability (see Chapter 13), where several good-quality trials—especially of risperidone—have received systematic reviews and led to approval by regulators. This evidence has sustained their use in treating irritability whatever the cause and whatever the psychiatric diagnosis.

Table 14.3 Considerations specific to individual second-generation antipsychotics

Drug	Receptor actions additional to generic	Use for control of irritability	Safety considerations
Risperidone, paliperidone and others	Generic; see text	Irritability in autism	Risperidone has lower risk for seizures than many antipsychotics
Quetiapine	H1 blocker Alpha-1 adrenoreceptor blockade Low D2-binding	Helpful actions on depression	Sedative Hypothyroidism Low rate of EPS Low rate of epilepsy Low rate of hyperprolactinaemia
Amisulpride (low dose)	Inhibits dopamine autoreceptors	Not approved for any purpose in USA (possibly helpful for negative symptoms)	Agitation
Amisulpride (high dose) (>400 mg)	Inhibits post-synaptic receptors Antagonizes 5HT-7 Little effect on 5HT-1A, -2A, C blockade	Possibly helpful for depression	Q–T interval prolonged
Aripiprazole	Partial dopamine agonist	Adjunctive in major depression Irritability in ASD	Less metabolic and endocrine risks than most antipsychotics; somewhat more EPS
Olanzapine	Multiple receptor antagonism including muscarinic M3	Weak evidence for value	High efficacy High rates of obesity, metabolic and endocrine problems

5HT, serotonin; EPS, extrapyramidal symptoms; ASD, autism spectrum disorders.

Antipsychotics also have a worrying profile of adverse effects in the large doses used for the treatment of psychiatric illnesses The first generation of antipsychotics (chlorpromazine being the standard) had notorious effects on the extrapyramidal motor system which may have been even more frequent, stigmatizing, and disabling for young patients. The second generation of antipsychotics (risperidone being the most widely used) have less propensity than first-generation drugs to alter motor control, but a higher rate of metabolic adverse effects: obesity, increases in blood levels of triglycerides, non-high-density lipoproteins, cholesterol, and glucose (which can even amount to Type II diabetes), and endocrine changes such as hyperprolactinaemia (which can result in inappropriate lactation for both sexes and polycystic ovaries and menstrual irregularities in girls and women). Constipation can become a serious problem in developmentally disabled children.

In low doses (up to 2 mg of risperidone) and for short periods (up to 3 months of continuous use) the benefits can sometimes outweigh the hazards for severely affected children whose lives are being harmed by their problems and who have not been helped by psychological measures. The balance of risk and benefit is more complex in situations where appropriate psychological help has not been given. The benefit is then reduced by the possibility that they could have improved without exposure to the risks of medication. Furthermore, ethical aspects have to be considered carefully when the main impact of the problem is on other people rather than the child. Other family members may then be getting the main benefit while the main risks are borne by the child or young person.

Hazards are proportional to blood levels, which are determined not only by dose level but also by metabolism in the liver. Different second-generation antipsychotics are broken down by different cytochrome isoenzymes. Interactions with other drugs and food substances which inhibit those enzymes (e.g. some antidepressants) or potentiate their action (e.g. some anticonvulsants) will therefore vary from drug to drug. Prescribers should generally use a small range of drugs that they know well and seek advice when a different one is needed.

Long-term use, beyond the 3-month limit, is occasionally justified when monitoring for possible hazards can be maintained and when there is clear evidence for little adverse effect and for major value—for instance being enabled to continue living at home when this is otherwise in jeopardy. There is a temptation to allow doses to drift up over time: as in any fluctuating disorder, exacerbations can be met with an increase of dose and periods of stability by 'leaving well alone'. We recommend monthly checks, including rating scales, with plans for dose reductions during periods of relative calm. Physical monitoring, including weight plotted on growth charts, can be done 3-monthly if the dose is low and not increasing.

Chapter 15

Future directions and a model for irritability

Irritability has sometimes been regarded in the past as a heterogeneous behavioural problem, occurring in most of the disorders of child mental health but without special significance for management. As we have reviewed across the different disorders we have been struck by the features that are consistent across conditions. Whether in ADHD, ODD, DMDD, or diffuse brain disorders, it presents as a disorder of mood. Its management presents similar difficulties across the variety of presentations. Clinicians can with reason regard it as a coherent dimension of disturbed emotional development, and include it accordingly in their therapeutic planning. Researchers can integrate it into the 'domains' of disorder that may be closer than diagnostic categories to the processes by which psychopathology develops.

These ways of thinking will call out new research. Indeed the gaps in our knowledge could usefully occupy the careers of several researchers for years to come. Clinically and practically, there are pressing needs to know more about the influences on persistence or remission of enduring angry states. Therapeutic trials for children with severe and chronic irritability are needed. Conceptually, too, we need advances to be made. Here we will highlight what we see as the main directions of irritability research for the future.

Irritability, the threat circuit, and other emotions

In Chapter 6 we discussed how activation of a brain network of threat, encompassing the amygdala, hypothalamus, and periaqueductal grey, may also underlie irritability. This brain circuit is thought to provide an evolutionarily conserved substrate for responding to threatening stimuli. It is suggested that environmental contingencies, particularly whether escape is possible or not, determine behavioural and feeling outcome. In the absence of the possibility of escape, reactive aggression rather than fearful escape is to be expected.

This is a very attractive model which has not yet been explicitly tested in animals or in humans. It should be relatively straightforward to test. Our hypothesis is that, within one and the same individual, environmental contingencies should determine the behaviour and the feelings that characterize the response. The question then will be which brain regions calculate the environmental contingencies. Following Rolls and others, we would expect the orbitofrontal cortex to play a key role, at least for value estimation, and the anterior cingulate cortex to be involved in conflict monitoring. However, it will be key to determine whether distinguishing between potential outcomes follows a distinct topography and how this may map onto behaviours and feelings. Conducting such experiments will be of service to the field of irritability, but it could also resolve some of the long-standing conundrums about the physiological substrates of phenomenologically distinct emotions.

Having tested this, the question will be how one accounts for interindividual differences: some people are far more prone to irritability than they are to fearful withdrawal. Our hypothesis is that, at least in part, this will be determined by prior experience (including social learning). Again this is testable in both animals and humans, and experimental set-ups with priming of subjects could provide important clues. Again, a key question will be to distinguish between brain areas—presumably autobiographical information retrieved from the hippocampal formation. We expect language—in the form of elaborations and narratives attached to events—to have a powerful influence on emotion regulation. Evidently, conducting such experiments could provide treatment targets for psychological treatment and possibly innovative interventions such as neurofeedback.

Irritability: duration and mood state

The previous section focused on irritability as a response to an event. However, common experience suggests that irritability may set in pretty much out of the blue or at least without an apparent precipitant. Many patients describe that they wake up and feel irritable without quite knowing why. Moreover, patients describe such a state of irritability to be long-lasting (minutes, hours, or days). These long-lasting moods are very hard (and ethically problematic) to induce in humans in the laboratory. However, until we have started studying these phenomena in more depth we will not know how close phasic irritability (the response to a threat cue) is to persistent or tonic irritability. Children with long-standing irritability (e.g. those scoring 'a lot' on items like 'my irritability lasts for the whole day') are far fewer in number than those who have tantrums and seem more impaired. It remains unclear whether they are a distinct group in pathophysiological terms. From a neuroscience point of view, the gap in our understanding about what causes longer-standing mood states is very wide. It is unclear what brain mechanisms underlie the chronicity of a mood. Irritability seems a much easier target for probing this important problem—certainly using animal frustration moments in the first instance—before generalizing it to include other moods such as depression or mania. Investigating the role of neurotransmitters—and understanding the functional alterations they cause—will be key. In this respect, variations of the depletion experiments using functional imaging in animals and humans should be a good way forward. Insights from such experiments could form the most fruitful ground for drug development in the mood disorders.

Irritability: one or more?

The evidence so far suggests that irritability is a dimension that cuts across disorders. It is correlated with other dimensions of psychopathology (e.g. anxiety), but separable from them. Moreover, it seems to follow its own developmental course with considerable stability across time. In addition, irritability predicts future psychopathology and impairment independently of the presence of other disorders, as we have discussed. It remains unclear whether the irritability that one encounters in, say, ADHD has the same aetiology as that in a child with depression. To use an analogy, it is reasonable to assume that the aetiological processes involved in fear in a phobic disorder and in someone with depression are the same or very similar (although the content of the fear, that which is feared, may be different). However, a counterexample is attention and concentration: children with ADHD are unable to concentrate, probably for different reasons from the ones that make it hard for those with generalized anxiety disorder to concentrate. Where would irritability fall? As mentioned, at present it seems that irritability is a dimension that cuts across disorders. But this may be because our measurement of irritability is too crude. Moreover, the fact that irritability improves with a variety of treatments—often specific to underlying disorders—seems to suggest at least some common aetiological mechanisms. We recommend the following research directions to address this key question: first, qualitative reports of parents and children across disorders; secondly, contextual measurement; thirdly, use of genetically informative designs; finally, experimental and imaging designs across different conditions.

Appendix

A scale to measure irritability

Please follow this link for more information on the questionnaires and translation into other languages: <http://www.kcl.ac.uk/ioppn/depts/cap/research/moodlab/ari.aspx>

ARI-*P*

Name of participant: Age:

For each item, please mark the box for Not True, Somewhat True or Certainly True.

In the *last six months* and compared to others of the same age, how well does each of the following statements describe the behavior/feelings of your child? Please try to answer all questions.

	NOT TRUE	SOMEWHAT TRUE	CERTAINLY TRUE
Is easily annoyed by others	☐	☐	☐
Often loses his/her temper	☐	☐	☐
Stays angry for a long time	☐	☐	☐
Is angry most of the time	☐	☐	☐
Gets angry frequently	☐	☐	☐
Loses temper easily	☐	☐	☐
Overall, *irritability* causes him/her problems	☐	☐	☐

THANK YOU VERY MUCH FOR YOUR HELP.

ARI-*S*

Name of participant: Age:

For each item, please mark the box for Not True, Somewhat True or Certainly True.

In the *last six months* and compared to others of the same age, how well does each of the following statements describe your behavior/feelings? Please try to answer all questions.

	NOT TRUE	SOMEWHAT TRUE	CERTAINLY TRUE
I am easily annoyed by others	☐	☐	☐
I often lose my temper	☐	☐	☐
I stay angry for a long time	☐	☐	☐
I am angry most of the time	☐	☐	☐
I get angry frequently	☐	☐	☐
I lose my temper easily	☐	☐	☐
Overall, my *irritability* causes me problems.	☐	☐	☐

THANK YOU VERY MUCH FOR YOUR HELP

References

Abraham, K. 1911. *Notes on the psycho-analytical investigation and treatment of manic-depressive insanity and allied conditions*. London: Leonard and Virginia Woolf at the Hogarth Press and Institute of Psychoanalysis.

Achenbach, T. M. 1991. *Manual for the child behaviour checklist 4–18 and 1991 profile*. Burlington: University of Vermont, Department of Psychiatry.

Adamson, L. B., et al. 2003. The still face: a history of a shared experimental paradigm. *Infancy*, 4, 451–73.

Adleman, N. E., et al. 2011. Neural correlates of reversal learning in severe mood dysregulation and pediatric bipolar disorder. *J Am Acad Child Adolesc Psychiatry*, 50, 1173–85.e2.

Aebi, M., et al. 2010. Predictability of oppositional defiant disorder and symptom dimensions in children and adolescents with ADHD combined type. *Psychol Med*, 40, 2089–100.

Aebi, M., et al. 2012. The use of the development and well-being assessment (DAWBA) in clinical practice: a randomized trial. *Eur Child Adolesc Psychiatry*, 21, 559–67.

Aman, M. G., et al. 1985. The aberrant behavior checklist: a behavior rating scale for the assessment of treatment effects. *Am J Ment Defic*, 89, 485–91.

Aman, M. G., et al. 2002. Double-blind, placebo-controlled study of risperidone for the treatment of disruptive behaviors in children with subaverage intelligence. *Am J Psychiatry*, 159, 1337–46.

Aman, M. G., et al. 2004. Risperidone effects in the presence/absence of psychostimulant medicine in children with ADHD, other disruptive behavior disorders, and subaverage IQ. *J Child Adolesc Psychopharmacol*, 14, 243–54.

Aman, M. G., et al. 2005. Acute and long-term safety and tolerability of risperidone in children with autism. *J Child Adolesc Psychopharmacol*, 15, 869–84.

Aman, M. G., et al. 2009. Medication and parent training in children with pervasive developmental disorders and serious behavior problems: results from a randomized clinical trial. *J Am Acad Child Adolesc Psychiatry*, 48, 1143–54.

Ambrosini, P. J., et al. 2013. Attention deficit hyperactivity disorder characteristics: II. Clinical correlates of irritable mood. *J Affect Disord*, 145, 70–6.

Angold, A., et al. 1995a. A test–retest reliability study of child-reported psychiatric symptoms and diagnoses using the Child and Adolescent Psychiatric Assessment (CAPA-C). *Psychol Med*, 25, 755–62.

Angold, A., et al. 1995b. The Child and Adolescent Psychiatric Assessment (CAPA). *Psychol Med*, 25, 739–53.

Angold, A., et al. 1999. Comorbidity. *J Child Psychol Psychiatry*, 40, 57–87.

American Psychiatric Association 2000. *Diagnostic and statistical manual of mental disorders: DSM-IV-TR*. Washington, DC: American Psychiatric Press.

American Psychiatric Association 2013. *Diagnostic and statistical manual of mental disorders: DSM-5*. Washington, DC: American Psychiatric Association.

Averill, J. R. 1982. *Anger and aggression: An essay on emotion*. New York: Springer.

Baguley, I. J., et al. 2006. Aggressive behavior following traumatic brain injury: how common is common? *J Head Trauma Rehabil*, 21, 45–56.

Bandura, A. 1973. *Aggression: A social learning analysis*. Upper Saddle River, NJ: Prentice Hall.

Bank, L., et al. 1991. A comparative evaluation of parent-training interventions for families of chronic delinquents. *J Abnorm Child Psychol*, 19, 15–33.

Barkley, R. A., et al. 2010. The unique contribution of emotional impulsiveness to impairment in major life activities in hyperactive children as adults. *J Am Acad Child Adolesc Psychiatry*, 49, 503–13.

Barnhart, R. K. (ed.) 1988. Irritate. *Chambers dictionary of etymology*. Edinburgh: Chambers.

Barrett, L. F. 2011. Was Darwin wrong about emotional expressions? *Curr Dir Psychol Sci*, 20, 400–6.

Barzman, D. H., et al. 2004. The effectiveness and tolerability of aripiprazole for pediatric bipolar disorders: a retrospective chart review. *J Child Adolesc Psychopharmacol*, 14, 593–600.

Bates, J. E., et al. 1998. Interaction of temperamental resistance to control and restrictive parenting in the development of externalizing behavior. *Dev Psychol*, 34, 982–95.

Bear, G. G., et al. 2009. Shame, guilt, blaming, and anger: differences between children in Japan and the US. *Motiv Emotion*, 33, 229–38.

Beesdo, K., et al. 2009. Common and distinct amygdala-function perturbations in depressed vs anxious adolescents. *Arch Gen Psychiatry*, 66, 275–85.

Behrmann, M., et al. 2004. Parietal cortex and attention. *Curr Opin Neurobiol*, 14, 212–17.

Biederman, J. 2006. The evolving face of pediatric mania. *Biol Psychiatry*, 60, 901.

Biederman, J., et al. 2005. Open-label, 8-week trial of olanzapine and risperidone for the treatment of bipolar disorder in preschool-age children. *Biol Psychiatry*, 58, 589–94.

Biederman, J., et al. 2007. A prospective open-label treatment trial of ziprasidone monotherapy in children and adolescents with bipolar disorder. *Bipolar Disord*, 9, 888–94.

Birmaher, B., et al. 2009. Four-year longitudinal course of children and adolescents with bipolar spectrum disorders: the Course and Outcome of Bipolar Youth (COBY) study. *Am J Psychiatry*, 166, 795–804.

Blader, J. C., et al. 2007. Increased rates of bipolar disorder diagnoses among U.S. child, adolescent, and adult inpatients, 1996–2004. *Biol Psychiatry*, 62, 107.

Blader, J. C., et al. 2009. Adjunctive divalproex versus placebo for children with ADHD and aggression refractory to stimulant monotherapy. *Am J Psychiatry*, 166, 1392–401.

Blair, R. J. 2012. Considering anger from a cognitive neuroscience perspective. *Wiley Interdiscip Rev. Cogn Sci*, 3, 65–74.

Blair, R. J. 2013. The neurobiology of psychopathic traits in youths. *Nat Rev Neurosci*, 14, 786–99.

Bleuler, E. 1983. *Lehrbuch der Psychiatrie*. Berlin: Springer Verlag.

Borke, H., et al. 1972. Perception of emotional responses to social interactions by Chinese and American children. *J Cross-Cult Psychol*, 3, 309–14.

Boylan, K., et al. 2007. Comorbidity of internalizing disorders in children with oppositional defiant disorder. *Eur Child Adolesc Psychiatry*, 16, 484–94.

Bradley, E., et al. 2006. Episodic psychiatric disorders in teenagers with learning disabilities with and without autism. *Br J Psychiatry*, 189, 361–6.

Brent, D., et al. 2008. Switching to another SSRI or to venlafaxine with or without cognitive behavioral therapy for adolescents with SSRI-resistant depression: the TORDIA randomized controlled trial. *J Am Med Assoc*, 299, 901–13.

Brooks, B. R., et al. 2004. Treatment of pseudobulbar affect in ALS with dextromethorphan/quinidine: a randomized trial. *Neurology*, 63, 1364–70.

Brotman, M. A., et al. 2006. Prevalence, clinical correlates, and longitudinal course of severe mood dysregulation in children. *Biol Psychiatry*, 60, 991–7.

Brotman, M. A., et al. 2007. Parental diagnoses in youth with narrow phenotype bipolar disorder or severe mood dysregulation. *Am J Psychiatry*, 164, 1238–41.

Brotman, M. A., et al. 2010. Amygdala activation during emotion processing of neutral faces in children with severe mood dysregulation versus ADHD or bipolar disorder. *Am J Psychiatry*, 167, 61–9.

Brown, J., et al. 2009. Selective serotonin reuptake inhibitors for premenstrual syndrome. *Cochrane Database Syst Rev*, (2):CD001396.

Budhani, S., et al. 2007. Neural correlates of response reversal: considering acquisition. *NeuroImage*, 34, 1754–65.

Burke, J. D. 2012. An affective dimension within oppositional defiant disorder symptoms among boys: personality and psychopathology outcomes into early adulthood. *J Child Psychol Psychiatry*, 53, 1176–83.

Burke, J. D., et al. 2010. Dimensions of oppositional defiant disorder as predictors of depression and conduct disorder in preadolescent girls. *J Am Acad Child Adolesc Psychiatry*, 49, 484–92.

Burton, R. 1932. Symptoms or signs in the mind. In: Jackson, H. (ed.) *The anatomy of melancholy*. Totowa, NJ: J. M. Dent & Sons Ltd.

Bushman, B. J. & Anderson, C. A. 2001. Is it time to pull the plug on hostile versus instrumental aggression dichotomy? *Psychol Rev*, 108, 273–9.

Buss, K. A. & Goldsmith, H. H. 1998. Fear and anger regulation in infancy: effects on the temporal dynamics of affective expression. *Child Dev*, 69, 359–74.

Calabrese, J. R., et al. 2005. A randomized, double-blind, placebo-controlled trial of quetiapine in the treatment of bipolar I or II depression. *Am J Psychiatry*, 162, 1351–60.

Calkins, S. D., et al. 2002. Frustration in infancy: implications for emotion regulation, physiological processes, and temperament. Infancy, 3, 175–97.

Canitano, R., et al. 2011. Psychopharmacology in autism: an update. *Prog Neuropsychopharmacol Biol Psychiatry*, 35, 18–28.

Capaldi, D. M. 1992. Co-occurrence of conduct problems and depressive symptoms in early adolescent boys: II. A 2-year follow-up at Grade 8. *Dev Psychopathol*, 4, 125–44.

Carr, E. G., et al. 2002. Positive behavior support: evolution of an applied science. *J Positive Behav Intervent*, 4, 4–16.

Caspi, A., et al. 1996. Behavioral observations at age 3 years predict adult psychiatric disorders. Longitudinal evidence from a birth cohort. *Arch Gen Psychiatry*, 53, 1033–9.

Caspi, A., et al. 2002. Role of genotype in the cycle of violence in maltreated children. *Science*, 297, 851–4.

Caspi, A., et al. 2004. Maternal expressed emotion predicts children's antisocial behavior problems: using monozygotic-twin differences to identify environmental effects on behavioral development. *Dev Psychol*, 40, 149–61.

Chadwick, O., et al. 2000. Factors affecting the risk of behaviour problems in children with severe intellectual disability. *J Intellect Disabil Res*, 44, 108–23.

Chambers, W. J., et al. 1985. The assessment of affective disorders in children and adolescents by semistructured interview. Test–retest reliability of the schedule for affective disorders and schizophrenia for school-age children, present episode version. *Arch Gen Psychiatry*, 42, 696–702.

Charach, A., et al. 2013. Interventions for preschool children at high risk for ADHD: a comparative effectiveness review. *Pediatrics*, 131, e1584–604.

Cipriani, A., et al. 2011. Comparative efficacy and acceptability of antimanic drugs in acute mania: a multiple-treatments meta-analysis. *Lancet*, 378, 1306–15.

Clin J. Psychiatry. 2013. Jan;74(1):e100–9. doi: 10.4088/JCP.11m07424. Efficacy and safety of quetiapine in children and adolescents with mania associated with bipolar I disorder: a 3-week, double-blind, placebo-controlled trial. Pathak S1, Findling RL, Earley WR, Acevedo LD, Stankowski J, Delbello MP.

Cloninger, C. R., et al. 1993. A psychobiological model of temperament and character. *Arch Gen Psychiatry*, 50, 975–90.

Coccaro, E. F., et al. 1997. Heritability of aggression and irritability: a twin study of the Buss–Durkee aggression scales in adult male subjects. *Biol Psychiatry*, 41, 273–84.

Cole, P. M., et al. 2003. Mutual emotion regulation and the stability of conduct problems between preschool and early school age. *Dev Psychopathol*, 15, 1–18.

Cole, P. M., et al. 2006. Cultural variations in the socialization of young children's anger and shame. *Child Dev*, 77, 1237–51.

Colom, F., et al. 2003. A randomized trial on the efficacy of group psychoeducation in the prophylaxis of recurrences in bipolar patients whose disease is in remission. *Arch Gen Psychiatry*, 60, 402–7.

Connor, D. F., et al. 2002. Psychopharmacology and aggression. I: A meta-analysis of stimulant effects on overt/covert aggression-related behaviors in ADHD. *J Am Acad Child Adolesc Psychiatry*, 41, 253–61.

Consoli, A., et al. 2007. Treatments in child and adolescent bipolar disorders. *Eur Child Adolesc Psychiatry*, 16, 187–98.

Copeland, W., et al. 2009. Configurations of common childhood psychosocial risk factors. *J Child Psychol Psychiatry*, 50, 451–9.

Copeland, W. E., et al. 2013. Prevalence, comorbidity, and correlates of DSM-5 proposed disruptive mood dysregulation disorder. *Am J Psychiatry*, 170, 173–9.

Correll, C. U., et al. 2010. Antipsychotic and mood stabilizer efficacy and tolerability in pediatric and adult patients with bipolar I mania: a comparative analysis of acute, randomized, placebo-controlled trials. *Bipolar Disord*, 12, 116–41.

Cortese, S., et al. 2013. Practitioner review: current best practice in the management of adverse events during treatment with ADHD medications in children and adolescents. *J Child Psychol Psychiatry*, 54, 227–46.

Costello, E. J., et al. 1996. The Great Smoky Mountains Study of Youth. Goals, design, methods, and the prevalence of DSM-III-R disorders. *Arch Gen Psychiatry*, 53, 1129–36.

Couppis, M. H. & Kennedy, C. H. 2008. The rewarding effect of aggression is reduced by nucleus accumbens dopamine receptor antagonism in mice. *Psychopharmacology*, 197, 449–56.

Cummings, E. M., et al. 1981. Young children's responses to expressions of anger and affection by others in the family. *Child Dev*, 52, 1274–82.

Dailey, L. F., et al. 2005. Recidivism in medication-noncompliant serious juvenile offenders with bipolar disorder. *J Clin Psychiatry*, 66, 477–84.

Davis, M., et al. 2010. Phasic vs sustained fear in rats and humans: role of the extended amygdala in fear vs anxiety. *Neuropsychopharmacology*, 35, 105–35.

Dayu, L., et al. 2011. Functional identification of an aggression locus in the mouse hypothalamus. *Nature*, 470, 221–6.

Deater-Deckard, K., et al. 2007. Anger/frustration, task persistence, and conduct problems in childhood: a behavioral genetic analysis. *J Child Psychol Psychiatry*, 48, 80–7.

De Boer, S. F., et al. 2005. 5-HT1A and 5-HT1B receptor agonists and aggression: A pharmacological challenge of the serotonin deficiency hypothesis. *Eur J Pharmacol*, 526, 125–39.

Deffenbacher, J., et al. 2000. *Overcoming situational and general anger: Therapist protocol*. Oakland, CA: New Harbinger Publications Inc.

De Hert, M., et al. 2011. Metabolic and endocrine adverse effects of second-generation antipsychotics in children and adolescents: a systematic review of randomized, placebo controlled trials and guidelines for clinical practice. *Eur Psychiatry*, 26, 144–58.

Delbello, M. P., et al. 2002. A double-blind, randomized, placebo-controlled study of quetiapine as adjunctive treatment for adolescent mania. *J Am Acad Child Adolesc Psychiatry*, 41, 1216–23.

Delbello, M. P., et al. 2006. A double-blind randomized pilot study comparing quetiapine and divalproex for adolescent mania. *J Am Acad Child Adolesc Psychiatry*, 45, 305–13.

Deltito, J. A., et al. 1998. Naturalistic experience with the use of divalproex sodium on an in-patient unit for adolescent psychiatric patients. *Acta Psychiatr Scand*, 97, 236–40.

Deveney, C. M., et al. 2013. Neural mechanisms of frustration in chronically irritable children. *Am J Psychiatry*, 170, 1186–94.

Dickstein, D. P., et al. 2007. Cognitive flexibility in phenotypes of pediatric bipolar disorder. *J Am Acad Child Adolesc Psychiatry*, 46, 341–55.

Dickstein, D. P., et al. 2009. Randomized double-blind placebo-controlled trial of lithium in youths with severe mood dysregulation. *J Child Adolesc Psychopharmacol*, 19, 61–73.

Diener, M. L., et al. 1999. Behavioral strategies for emotion regulation in toddlers: associations with maternal involvement and emotional expressions. *Infant Behav Dev*, 22, 569–83.

Dodds, C. M., et al. 2011. Dissociating inhibition, attention, and response control in the frontoparietal network using functional magnetic resonance imaging. *Cereb Cortex*, 21, 1155–65.

Dodge, K. A., et al. 1987. Hostile attributional biases among aggressive boys are exacerbated under conditions of threats to the self. *Child Dev*, 58, 213–24.

Domizio, S., et al. 1993. Anti-epileptic therapy and behaviour disturbances in children. *Child Nerv Syst*, 9, 272–4.

Donovan, S. J., et al. 2000. Divalproex treatment for youth with explosive temper and mood lability: a double-blind, placebo-controlled crossover design. *Am J Psychiatry*, 157, 818–20.

Drabick, D. A., et al. 2012. Deconstructing oppositional defiant disorder: clinic-based evidence for an anger/irritability phenotype. *J Am Acad Child Adolesc Psychiatry*, 51, 384–93.

Duke, A. A., et al. 2013. Revisiting the serotonin–aggression relation in humans: a meta-analysis. *Psychol Bull*, 139, 1148–72.

Eisenberg, N. 2000. Emotion, regulation, and moral development. *Annu Rev Psychol*, 51, 665–97.

Eisenberg, N., et al. 1994. The relations of emotionality and regulation to children's anger-related reactions. *Child Dev*, 65, 109–28.

Ekman, P., et al. 2011. What is meant by calling emotions basic? *Emotion Rev*, 3, 364–70.

Elbe, D., et al. 2012. Review of the pharmacotherapy of irritability of autism. *J Can Acad Child Adolesc Psychiatry*, 21, 130–46.

Eley, T. C. 1997. General genes: a new theme in developmental psychopathology. *Curr Direct Psychol Sci*, 6, 90–5.

Esser, G., et al. 1990. Epidemiology and course of psychiatric disorders in school-age children—results of a longitudinal study. *J Child Psychol Psychiatry*, 31, 243–63.

Fabes, R. A. & Eisenberg, N. (1992). Young children's coping with interpersonal anger. *Child Dev*, 63, 116–28.

Fava, M., et al. 2010. The importance of irritability as a symptom of major depressive disorder: results from the National Comorbidity Survey Replication. *Mol Psychiatry*, 15, 856–67.

FDA 2008 *Antiepileptic drugs and suicidality*. URL: <http://www.fda.gov/downloads/Drugs/DrugSafety/PostmarketDrugSafetyInformationforPatientsandProviders/UCM192556.pdf>

Feindler, E. L., et al. 1986. *Adolescent anger control: Cognitive-behavioral techniques*. New York: Pergamon Press.

Feldman, R., et al. 1999. Mother–infant affect synchrony as an antecedent of the emergence of self-control. *Dev Psychol*, 35, 223–31.

Fernández de la Cruz, L., Simonoff, E., McGough, J. J., Halperin, J.M., Arnold, L. E., Stringaris, A. 2015. Treatment of children with attention-deficit/hyperactivity disorder (ADHD) and irritability: results from the multimodal treatment study of children with ADHD (MTA). *J Am Acad Child Adolesc Psychiatry*, 54(1), 62–70.e3. doi:10.1016/j.jaac.2014.10.006.

Ferrin, M., et al. 2011. Child and caregiver issues in the treatment of attention deficit–hyperactivity disorder: education, adherence and treatment choice. *Future Neurol*, 6, 399–413.

Findling, R. L., et al. 2003. Combination lithium and divalproex sodium in pediatric bipolarity. *J Am Acad Child Adolesc Psychiatry*, 42, 895–901.

Findling, R. L., et al. 2004. Long-term, open-label study of risperidone in children with severe disruptive behaviors and below-average IQ. *Am J Psychiatry*, 161, 677–84.

Findling, R. L., et al. 2005. Double-blind 18-month trial of lithium versus divalproex maintenance treatment in pediatric bipolar disorder. *J Am Acad Child Adolesc Psychiatry*, 44, 409–17.

Findling, R. L., et al. 2009. Acute treatment of pediatric bipolar I disorder, manic or mixed episode, with aripiprazole: a randomized, double-blind, placebo-controlled study. *J Clin Psychiatry*, 70, 1441–51.

Fleminger, S., et al. 2006. Pharmacological management for agitation and aggression in people with acquired brain injury. *Cochrane Database Syst Rev*, (4):CD003299.

Fombonne, E. 1994. The Chartres Study: I. Prevalence of psychiatric disorders among French school-age children. *Br J Psychiatry*, 164, 69–79.

Ford, T., et al. 2003. The British Child and Adolescent Mental Health Survey 1999: the prevalence of DSM-IV disorders. *J Am Acad Child Adolesc Psychiatry*, 42, 1203–11.

Frankenhaeuser, M. 1971. Behavior and circulating catecholamines. *Brain Res*, 31, 241–62.

Frazier, J. A., et al. 2001. A prospective open-label treatment trial of olanzapine monotherapy in children and adolescents with bipolar disorder. *J Child Adolesc Psychopharmacol*, 11, 239–50.

Freud, S. 1915. *Trauer und Melancholie*. Frankfurt: Fischer Taschenbuch Verlag.

Fristad, M. A. 2006. Psychoeducational treatment for school-aged children with bipolar disorder. *Dev Psychopathol*, 18, 1289–306.

Gagne, J. R. & Hill Goldsmith, H. 2011. A longitudinal analysis of anger and inhibitory control in twins from 12 to 36 months of age. *Dev Sci*, 14, 112–24.

Geller, B., et al. 1998. Prepubertal and early adolescent bipolarity differentiate from ADHD by manic symptoms, grandiose delusions, ultra-rapid or ultradian cycling. *J Affect Disord*, 51, 81.

Geller, B., et al. 2002. DSM-IV mania symptoms in a prepubertal and early adolescent bipolar disorder phenotype compared to attention-deficit hyperactive and normal controls. *J Child Adolesc Psychopharmacol*, 12, 11–25.

Goodman, R. 1997. The Strengths and Difficulties Questionnaire: a research note. *J Child Psychol Psychiatry*, 38, 581–6.

Goodman, R., et al. 2000. The Development and Well-Being Assessment: description and initial validation of an integrated assessment of child and adolescent psychopathology. *J Child Psychol Psychiatry*, 41, 645–55.

Goodwin, F. K., et al. 2007. Epidemiology. In: *Manic-depressive illness*, pp. 155–86. Oxford: Oxford University Press.

van Goozen, S. H., et al. 1998. Salivary cortisol and cardiovascular activity during stress in oppositional-defiant disorder boys and normal controls. *Biol Psychiatry*, 43, 531–9.

Haas, M., et al. 2009. Risperidone for the treatment of acute mania in children and adolescents with bipolar disorder: a randomized, double-blind, placebo-controlled study. *Bipolar Disord*, 11, 687–700.

Hagino, O. R., et al. 1995. Untoward effects of lithium treatment in children aged four through six years. *J Am Acad Child Adolesc Psychiatry*, 34, 1584–90.

Haller, J. 2013. The neurobiology of abnormal manifestations of aggression—a review of hypothalamic mechanisms in cats, rodents, and humans. *Brain Res Bull*, 93, 97–109.

Hardan, A. Y., et al. 2012. A randomized controlled pilot trial of oral *N*-acetylcysteine in children with autism. *Biol Psychiatry*, 71, 956–61.

Harris, W. V. 2002. *Restraining rage: The ideology of anger control in classical antiquity*. Cambridge, MA: Harvard University Press.

Hay, D. F., et al. 2011. Known risk factors for violence predict 12-month-old infants' aggressiveness with peers. *Psychol Sci*, 22, 1205–11.

Hellings, J.A., et al. 2006. A crossover study of risperidone in children, adolescents and adults with mental retardation. *J Autism Dev Disord*, 36, 401–11.

Henry, C. A., et al. 2003. Long-term outcome with divalproex in children and adolescents with bipolar disorder. *J Child Adolesc Psychopharmacol*, 13, 523–9.

Herrmann, D. S., et al. 2003. Anger and aggression management in young adolescents: an experimental validation of the SCARE program. *Educ Treat Children*, 26, 273–302.

Hesdorffer, D. C., et al. 2004. ADHD as a risk factor for incident unprovoked seizures and epilepsy in children. *Arch Gen Psychiatry*, 61, 731–6.

Ho, T. P., et al. 1996. Help-seeking behaviours among child psychiatric clinic attenders in Hong Kong. *Soc Psychiatry Psychiatr Epidemiol*, 31, 292–8.

Hollander, E., et al. 2006. A double-blind placebo-controlled pilot study of olanzapine in childhood/adolescent pervasive developmental disorder. *J Child Adolesc Psychopharmacol*, 16, 541–8.

Hollander, E., et al. 2010. Divalproex sodium vs placebo for the treatment of irritability in children and adolescents with autism spectrum disorders. *Neuropsychopharmacology*, 35, 990–8.

Howlin, P., et al. 2009. Systematic review of early intensive behavioral interventions for children with autism. *Am J Intellect Dev Disabil*, 114, 23–41.

Hunt, J., et al. 2009. Irritability without elation in a large bipolar youth sample: frequency and clinical description. *J Am Acad Child Adolesc Psychiatry*, 48, 730–9.

Izard, C. E., et al. 1995. The ontogeny and significance of infants' facial expressions in the first 9 months of life. *Dev Psychol*, 31, 997–1013.

Jack, R. E., et al. 2012. Facial expressions of emotion are not culturally universal. *Proc Natl Acad Sci USA*, 109, 7241–4.

Jones, A. P., et al. 2009. Amygdala hypoactivity to fearful faces in boys with conduct problems and callous-unemotional traits. *Am J Psychiatry*, 166, 95–102.

Jope, R. S. 1999. Anti-bipolar therapy: mechanism of action of lithium. *Mol Psychiatry*, 4, 117–28.

Judd, L. L., et al. 2013. Overt irritability/anger in unipolar major depressive episodes: past and current characteristics and implications for long-term course. *JAMA Psychiatry*, 70, 1171–80.

Kafantaris, V., et al. 2003. Lithium treatment of acute mania in adolescents: a large open trial. *J Am Acad Child Adolesc Psychiatry*, 42, 1038–45.

Kafantaris, V., et al. 2004. Lithium treatment of acute mania in adolescents: a placebo-controlled discontinuation study. *J Am Acad Child Adolesc Psychiatry*, 43, 984–93.

Kagan, J. 2004. *What is emotion?* New Haven, CT: Yale University Press.

Keltikangas-Jarvinen, L., et al. 2009. Dopamine and serotonin systems modify environmental effects on human behavior: a review. *Scand J Psychol*, 50, 574–82.

Ketter, T. A., et al. 2003. Physiological and pharmacological induction of affect. In: Davidson, J. R., Scherer, K. R., Goldsmith, H. H. (eds) *Handbook of affective sciences*, pp. 930–62. Oxford: Oxford University Press.

Kim-Cohen, J., et al. 2006. MAOA, maltreatment, and gene-environment interaction predicting children's mental health: new evidence and a meta-analysis. *Mol Psychiatry*, 11, 903–13.

Kochanska, G. 1997. Multiple pathways to conscience for children with different temperaments: from toddlerhood to age 5. *Dev Psychol*, 33, 228–40.

Kowatch, R. A., et al. 2003. Combination pharmacotherapy in children and adolescents with bipolar disorder. *Biol Psychiatry*, 53, 978–84.

Krebs, G., et al. 2013. Temper outbursts in paediatric obsessive–compulsive disorder and their association with depressed mood and treatment outcome. *J Child Psychol Psychiatry*, 54, 313–22.

Krieger, F. V., et al. 2011. An open-label trial of risperidone in children and adolescents with severe mood dysregulation. *J Child Adolesc Psychopharmacol*, 21, 237–43.

Krieger, F. V., et al. 2013. Dimensions of oppositionality in a Brazilian community sample: testing the DSM-5 proposal and etiological links. *J Am Acad Child Adolesc Psychiatry*, 52, 389–400.

Labarbera, J. D., et al. 1976. Four- and six-month-old infants' visual responses to joy, anger, and neutral expressions. *Child Dev*, 47, 535–8.

Lahey, B. B., et al. 1992. Oppositional defiant and conduct disorders: issues to be resolved for DSM-IV. *J Am Acad Child Adolesc Psychiatry*, 31, 539–46.

Lavigne, J. V., et al. 2001. Oppositional defiant disorder with onset in preschool years: longitudinal stability and pathways to other disorders. *J Am Acad Child Adolesc Psychiatry*, 40, 1393–400.

Lax Pericall, M. T., et al. 2014. Family function and its relationship to injury severity and psychiatric outcome in children with acquired brain injury: a systematized review. *Dev Med Child Neurol*, 56, 19–30.

Lecavalier, L. 2006. Behavioral and emotional problems in young people with pervasive developmental disorders: relative prevalence, effects of subject characteristics, and empirical classification. *J Autism Dev Disord*, 36, 1101–14.

Ledoux, J. E. 2000. Emotion circuits in the brain. *Annu Rev Neurosci*, 23, 155–84.

Leibenluft, E. 2011. Severe mood dysregulation, irritability, and the diagnostic boundaries of bipolar disorder in youths. *Am J Psychiatry*, 168, 129–42.

Leibenluft, E., et al. 2003. Defining clinical phenotypes of juvenile mania. *Am J Psychiatry*, 160, 430–7.

Leibenluft, E., et al. 2006. Chronic versus episodic irritability in youth: a community-based, longitudinal study of clinical and diagnostic associations. *J Child Adolesc Psychopharmacol*, 16, 456–66.

Leibenluft, E., et al. 2007. Neural circuitry engaged during unsuccessful motor inhibition in pediatric bipolar disorder. *Am J Psychiatry*, 164, 52–60.

Leigh, E., et al. 2012. Mood regulation in youth: research findings and clinical approaches to irritability and short-lived episodes of mania-like symptoms. *Curr Opin Psychiatry*, 25, 271–6.

Lench, H. C., et al. 2011. Discrete emotions predict changes in cognition, judgment, experience, behavior, and physiology: a meta-analysis of experimental emotion elicitations. *Psychol Bull*, 137, 834–55.

Lewinsohn, P. M., et al. 1993. Adolescent psychopathology: I. Prevalence and incidence of depression and other DSM-III-R disorders in high school students. *J Abnorm Psychol*, 102, 133–44.

Lewis, C. T. & Short, C. 1879. Irritabilis. In: Lewis, C. T. & Short, C. (eds) *A Latin dictionary. Founded upon Andrew's Edition of Freund's Latin Dictionary*. Oxford: Clarendon Press.

Lewis, M., et al. 2005. Infant emotional and cortisol responses to goal blockage. *Child Dev*, 76, 518–30.

Lindquist, K. A., et al. 2012. The brain basis of emotion: a meta-analytic review. *Behav Brain Sci*, 35, 121–43.

Lindquist, K. A., et al. 2013. The hundred-year emotion war: are emotions natural kinds or psychological constructions? Comment on Lench, Flores, and Bench (2011). *Psychol Bull*, 139, 255–63.

Liu, H. Y., et al. 2011. Pharmacologic treatments for pediatric bipolar disorder: a review and meta-analysis. *J Am Acad Child Adolesc Psychiatry*, 50, 749–62.

Lochman, J. E., et al. 2011. Cognitive-behavioral therapy for externalizing disorders in children and adolescents. *Child Adolesc Psychiatr Clin N Am*, 20, 305–18.

Loebel, A., et al. 2014. Lurasidone monotherapy in the treatment of bipolar I depression: a randomized, double-blind, placebo-controlled study. *Am J Psychiatry*, 171, 160–8.

Lövheim, H. 2012. A new three-dimensional model for emotions and monoamine neurotransmitters. *Med Hypoth*, 78, 341–8.

Luby, J., et al. 2006. Risperidone in preschool children with ASD: an investigation of safety and efficacy. J Child Adolesc Psychopharmacol, 16, 575–87.

McCann, D., et al. 2007. Food additives and hyperactive behaviour in 3-year-old and 8/9-year-old children in the community: a randomised, double-blinded, placebo-controlled trial. *Lancet*, 370, 1560–7.

McClellan, J., et al. 2007. Practice parameter for the assessment and treatment of children and adolescents with bipolar disorder. *J Am Acad Child Adolesc Psychiatry*, 46, 107–25.

McClintock, K., et al. 2003. Risk markers associated with challenging behaviours in people with intellectual disabilities: a meta-analytic study. *J Intellect Disabil Res*, 47, 405–16.

McCracken, J. T., et al. 2002. Risperidone in children with autism and serious behavioral problems. *N Engl J Med*, 347, 314–21.

McIntyre, R. S., et al. 2003. Valproate, bipolar disorder and polycystic ovarian syndrome. *Bipolar Disord*, 5, 28–35.

Maedgen, J. W., et al. 2000. Social functioning and emotional regulation in the attention deficit hyperactivity disorder subtypes. *J Clin Child Psychol*, 29, 30–42.

Malmquist, C. P. 1971. Depressions in childhood and adolescence. 1. *N Engl J Med*, 284, 887–93.

Manos, M. J., et al. 2011. Changes in emotions related to medication used to treat ADHD. Part I: literature review. *J Atten Disord*, 15, 101–12.

Marcus, R. N., et al. 2009. A placebo-controlled, fixed-dose study of aripiprazole in children and adolescents with irritability associated with autistic disorder. *J Am Acad Child Adolesc Psychiatry*, 48, 1110–19.

Masi, G., et al. 2002. Clozapine in adolescent inpatients with acute mania. *J Child Adolesc Psychopharmacol*, 12, 93–9.

Maughan, B., et al. 2013. Depression in childhood and adolescence. *J Can Acad Child Adolesc Psychiatry*, 22, 35–40.

Max, J. E., et al. 1997. Traumatic brain injury in children and adolescents: psychiatric disorders at two years. *J Am Acad Child Adolesc Psychiatry*, 36, 1278–85.

Mayes, S. D., et al. 2011. Anxiety, depression, and irritability in children with autism relative to other neuropsychiatric disorders and typical development. *Res Autism Spectrum Disord*, 5, 474–85.

Mendez, M. F., et al. 1993. Interictal violence in epilepsy. Relationship to behavior and seizure variables. *J Nerv Ment Dis*, 181, 566–9.

Merwood, A., et al. 2014. Genetic associations between the symptoms of attention-deficit/hyperactivity disorder and emotional lability in child and adolescent twins. *J Am Acad Child Adolesc Psychiatry*, 53, 209–20.e4.

Mesquita, B. & Frijda, N. H. 1992. Cultural variations in emotions: a review. *Psychol Bull*, 112, 179–204.

Mick, E., et al. 2005. Heterogeneity of irritability in attention-deficit/hyperactivity disorder subjects with and without mood disorders. *Biol Psychiatry*, 58, 576–82.

Mikita, N., et al. 2014. Irritability in boys with autism spectrum disorders: an investigation of physiological reactivity. *J Child Psychol Psychiatry*, (in press).

Miklowitz, D. J., et al. 2003. A randomized study of family-focused psychoeducation and pharmacotherapy in the outpatient management of bipolar disorder. *Arch Gen Psychiatry*, 60, 904–12.

Miklowitz, D. J., et al. 2008. Family-focused treatment for adolescents with bipolar disorder: results of a 2-year randomized trial. *Arch Gen Psychiatry*, 65, 1053–61.

Mobbs, D., et al. 2007. When fear is near: threat imminence elicits prefrontal-periaqueductal gray shifts in humans. *Science*, 317, 1079–83.

Mobbs, D., et al. 2010. Neural activity associated with monitoring the oscillating threat value of a tarantula. *Proc Natl Acad Sci USA*, 107, 20582–6.

Moreno, C., et al. 2007. National trends in the outpatient diagnosis and treatment of bipolar disorder in youth. *Arch Gen Psychiatry*, 64, 1032–9.

Morgan, S., et al. 2007. Antipsychotic drugs in children with autism. *Br Med J*, 334, 1069–70.

MTA 1999. A 14-month randomized clinical trial of treatment strategies for attention-deficit/hyperactivity disorder. The MTA Cooperative Group.

Multimodal Treatment Study of Children with ADHD. *Arch Gen Psychiatry*, 56, 1073–86.

Nagaraj, R., et al. 2006. Risperidone in children with autism: randomized, placebo-controlled, double-blind study. *J Child Neurol* 21, 450–5.

Narrow, W. E., et al. 2013. DSM-5 field trials in the United States and Canada, Part III: development and reliability testing of a cross-cutting symptom assessment for DSM-5. *Am J Psychiatry*, 170, 71–82.

NCHS 2006. *The international classification of diseases*, 9th revision, clinical modification. Washington, DC: Government Printing Office.

NICE (National Institute for Health and Care Excellence) 2006. Bipolar disorder. *The management of bipolar disorder in adults, children and adolescents, in primary and secondary care*. London: National Institute of Health and Care Excellence.

NICE (National Institute for Health and Care Excellence) 2007. Bipolar disorder: *The management of bipolar disorder in adults, children and adolescents, in primary and secondary care*. London: National Clinical Practice Guideline.

NICE (National Institute for Health and Care Excellence) 2008. *Attention deficit hyperactivity disorder: Diagnosis and management of ADHD in children, young people and adults*. NICE Clinical Guideline 72. URL: <http://www.nice.org.uk/CG72>

OED 2007. Irritability. *Shorter Oxford English dictionary*, 6th edn. Oxford: Oxford University Press.

Olfson, M., et al. 2006. National trends in the outpatient treatment of children and adolescents with antipsychotic drugs. *Arch Gen Psychiatry*, 63, 679–85.

Ortony, A., et al. 1990. What's basic about basic emotions? *Psychol Science*, 97, 315–31.

Owen, R., et al. 2009. Aripiprazole in the treatment of irritability in children and adolescents with autistic disorder. *Pediatrics*, 124, 1533–40.

Packard, M. G., et al. 2002. Learning and memory functions of the basal ganglia. *Annu Rev Neurosci*, 25, 563–93.

Pandina, G. J., et al. 2007. Risperidone improves behavioral symptoms in children with autism in a randomized, double-blind, placebo-controlled trial. *J Autism Dev Disord*, 37, 367–73.

Passarotti, A. M., et al. 2010. Emotion processing influences working memory circuits in pediatric bipolar disorder and attention-deficit/hyperactivity disorder. *J Am Acad Child Adolesc Psychiatry*, 49, 1064–80.

Pavuluri, M. N., et al. 2004. Open-label prospective trial of risperidone in combination with lithium or divalproex sodium in pediatric mania. *J Affect Disord*, 82, S103–S111.

Pavuluri, M. N., et al. 2010. Double-blind randomized trial of risperidone versus divalproex in pediatric bipolar disorder. *Bipolar Disord*, 12, 593–605.

Paykel, E. S. 1971. Classification of depressed patients: a cluster analysis derived grouping. *Br J Psychiatry*, 118, 275–88.

Perlis, R. H., et al. 2009. Irritability is associated with anxiety and greater severity, but not bipolar spectrum features, in major depressive disorder. *Acta Psychiatr Scand*, 119, 282–9.

Phillips, A. G., et al. 2003. Amygdalar control of the mesocorticolimbic dopamine system: parallel pathways to motivated behavior. *Neurosci Biobehav Rev*, 27, 543–54.

Phillips, M. L., et al. 2008. A neural model of voluntary and automatic emotion regulation: implications for understanding the pathophysiology and neurodevelopment of bipolar disorder. *Mol Psychiatry*, 13, 829–57.

Pickles, A., et al. 2003. Natural categories or fundamental dimensions: on carving nature at the joints and the rearticulation of psychopathology. *Dev Psychopathol*, 15, 529–51.

Pickles, A., et al. 2010. Predictors of suicidality across the life span: the Isle of Wight study. *Psychol Med*, 40, 1453–66.

Pilling, S., et al. 2013. Recognition, intervention, and management of antisocial behaviour and conduct disorders in children and young people: summary of NICE-SCIE guidance. *Br Med J*, 346, f1298.

Polanczyk, G., et al. 2007. The worldwide prevalence of ADHD: a systematic review and metaregression analysis. *Am J Psychiatry*, 164, 942–8.

Potegal, M., et al. 2003. Temper tantrums in young children: 2. Tantrum duration and temporal organization. *J Dev Behav Pediatr*, 24, 148–54.

Reddy, Y. C., et al. 2000. Juvenile bipolar disorder. *Acta Psychiatr Scand*, 102, 162–70.

Rodin, E. A. 1973. Psychomotor epilepsy and aggressive behavior. *Arch Gen Psychiatry*, 28, 210–13.

Rolls, E. T. 2007. *Emotion explained*. Oxford: Oxford University Press.

Rolls, E. T., et al. 1994. Emotion-related learning in patients with social and emotional changes associated with frontal lobe damage. *J Neurol, Neurosurg Psychiatry*, 57, 1518–24.

Rowe, K. S. & Rowe, K. J. 1994. Synthetic food coloring and behavior: a dose response effect in a double-blind, placebo-controlled, repeated-measures study. *J Pediatrics* 125, 691–8.

Rowe, R., et al. 2010. Developmental pathways in oppositional defiant disorder and conduct disorder. *J Abnorm Psychol*, 119, 726–38.

Ruhe, H. G., et al. 2007. Mood is indirectly related to serotonin, norepinephrine and dopamine levels in humans: a meta-analysis of monoamine depletion studies. *Mol Psychiatry*, 12, 331–59.

RUPPAN 2002. Research Units on Pediatric Psychopharmacology Autism Network. Risperidone in children with autism and serious behavioral problem. *N Engl J Med*, 347, 314–21.

Rutter, M. 2000. Genetic studies of autism: from the 1970s into the millennium. *J Abnorm Child Psychol*, 28, 3–14.

Rutter, M., et al. 1997. Integrating nature and nurture: implications of person-environment correlations and interactions for developmental psychopathology. *Dev Psychopathol*, 9, 335–64.

Sagvolden, T., et al. 2005. A dynamic developmental theory of attention-deficit/ hyperactivity disorder (ADHD) predominantly hyperactive/impulsive and combined subtypes. *Behav Brain Sci*, 28, 397–419.

Sano, K., et al, 1970. Results of stimulation and destruction of the posterior hypothalamus in man. *J Neurosurg*, 33, 689–707.

Savard, G., et al. 2003. Psychiatric aspects of patients with hypothalamic hamartoma and epilepsy. *Epileptic Disord*, 5, 229–34.

Scarpa, A. & Raine, A. 1997. Psychophysiology of anger and violent behavior. *Psychiat Clin N Am*, 20, 375–94.

Schachar, R., et al. 1987. Changes in family function and relationships in children who respond to methylphenidate. *J Am Acad Child Adolesc Psychiatry*, 26, 728–32.

Scheffer, R. E., et al. 2005. Randomized, placebo-controlled trial of mixed amphetamine salts for symptoms of comorbid ADHD in pediatric bipolar disorder after mood stabilization with divalproex sodium. *Am J Psychiatry*, 162, 58–64.

Scheres, A., et al. 2007. Ventral striatal hyporesponsiveness during reward anticipation in attention-deficit/hyperactivity disorder. *Biol Psychiatry*, 61, 720–4.

Schopler, E., et al. 1986. *The Childhood Autism Rating Scale (CARS): For diagnostic screening and classification of autism*. New York: Irvington.

Scott, S., et al. 2012. An experimental test of differential susceptibility to parenting among emotionally-dysregulated children in a randomized controlled trial for oppositional behavior. *J Child Psychol Psychiatry*, 53, 1184–93.

Seo, D., et al. 2008. Role of serotonin and dopamine system interactions in the neurobiology of impulsive aggression and its comorbidity with other clinical disorders. *Aggress Violent Behav*, 13, 383–95.

Shaffer, D., et al. 1975. Psychiatric outcome of localized head injury in children. *Ciba Found Symp*, 34, 191–213.

Shaw, P., et al. 2014. Emotion dysregulation in attention deficit hyperactivity disorder. *Am J Psychiatry*, 171, 276–93.

Shea, S., et al. 2004. Risperidone in the treatment of disruptive behavioral symptoms in children with autistic and other pervasive developmental disorders. *Pediatrics*, 114, e634–e641.

Siegel, A., et al. 1999. Neuropharmacology of brain-stimulation-evoked aggression. *Neurosci Biobehav Rev*, 23, 359–89.

Silva, H., et al. 2007. Serotonin transporter polymorphism and fluoxetine effect on impulsiveness and aggression in borderline personality disorder. *Actas Esp Psiquiatr*, 35, 387–92.

Silver, J. M., et al. 2011. *Textbook of traumatic brain injury*. Washington, DC: American Psychiatric Publishing Inc.

Simonoff, E., et al. 2008. Psychiatric disorders in children with autism spectrum disorders: prevalence, comorbidity, and associated factors in a population-derived sample. *J Am Acad Child Adolesc Psychiatry*, 47, 921–9.

Simonoff, E., et al. 2012. Severe mood problems in adolescents with autism spectrum disorder. *J Child Psychol Psychiatry*, 53, 1157–66.

Snyder, R., et al. 2002. Effects of risperidone on conduct and disruptive behavior disorders in children with subaverage IQs. *J Am Acad Child Adolesc Psychiatry*, 41, 1026–36.

Sobanski, E., et al. 2010. Emotional lability in children and adolescents with attention deficit/hyperactivity disorder (ADHD): clinical correlates and familial prevalence. *J Child Psychol Psychiatry*, 51, 915–23.

Sonuga-Barke, E. J., et al. 2013. Nonpharmacological interventions for ADHD: systematic review and meta-analyses of randomized controlled trials of dietary and psychological treatments. *Am J Psychiatry*, 170, 275–89.

Speltz, M. L., et al. 1999. Preschool boys with oppositional defiant disorder: clinical presentation and diagnostic change. *J Am Acad Child Adolesc Psychiatry*, 38, 838–45.

Spencer, T. J., et al. 2001. Parsing pediatric bipolar disorder from its associated comorbidity with the disruptive behavior disorders. *Biol Psychiatry*, 49, 1062–70.

Steinhausen, H. C., et al. 1998. Prevalence of child and adolescent psychiatric disorders: the Zurich Epidemiological Study. *Acta Psychiatr Scand*, 98, 262–71.

Stringaris, A. 2011. Irritability in children and adolescents: a challenge for DSM-5. *Eur Child Adolesc Psychiatry*, 20, 61–6.

Stringaris, A. in press. Emotion, emotion regulation and disorder: conceptual issues for clinicians and neuroscientists. In: Bishop, D., Pine, D., Scott, S., Stevenson, J., Taylor, E. & Thapar, A. (eds), *Rutter's child and adolescent psychiatry*, 6th edn. London: Wiley Blackwell.

Stringaris, A., et al. 2009a. Adult outcomes of youth irritability: a 20-year prospective community-based study. *Am J Psychiatry*, 166, 1048–54.

Stringaris, A., et al. 2009b. Longitudinal outcome of youth oppositionality: irritable, headstrong, and hurtful behaviors have distinctive predictions. *J Am Acad Child Adolesc Psychiatry*, 48, 404–12.

Stringaris, A., et al. 2009c. Mood lability and psychopathology in youth. *Psychol Med*, 39, 1237–45.

Stringaris, A., et al. 2009d. Three dimensions of oppositionality in youth. *J Child Psychol Psychiatry*, 50, 216–23.

Stringaris, A., et al. 2010a. Pediatric bipolar disorder versus severe mood dysregulation: risk for manic episodes on follow-up. *J Am Acad Child Adolesc Psychiatry*, 49, 397–405.

Stringaris, A., et al. 2010b. Youth meeting symptom and impairment criteria for mania-like episodes lasting less than four days: an epidemiological enquiry. *J Child Psychol Psychiatry*, 51, 31–8.

Stringaris, A., et al. 2012a. The Affective Reactivity Index: a concise irritability scale for clinical and research settings. *J Child Psychol Psychiatry*, 53, 1109–17.

Stringaris, A., et al. 2012b. Adolescent irritability: phenotypic associations and genetic links with depressed mood. *Am J Psychiatry* 169, 47–54.

Stringaris, A., et al. 2013. Irritable mood as a symptom of depression in youth: prevalence, developmental and clinical correlates in the Great Smoky Mountains Study. *J Am Acad Child Adolesec Psychiatry*, 52, 831–40.

Stringaris, A., et al. 2014. Developmental pathways from childhood conduct problems to young adult depression: findings from the ALSPAC cohort. *Br J Psychiatry*, 205, 17–23.

Strober, M., et al. 1995. Recovery and relapse in adolescents with bipolar affective illness: a five-year naturalistic, prospective follow-up. *J Am Acad Child Adolesc Psychiatry*, 34, 724–31.

Strober, M., et al. 1998. Early childhood attention deficit hyperactivity disorder predicts poorer response to acute lithium therapy in adolescent mania. *J Affect Disord*, 51, 145–51.

Strohle, A., et al. 2008. Reward anticipation and outcomes in adult males with attention-deficit/hyperactivity disorder. *NeuroImage*, 39, 966–72.

Sukhodolsky, D. G., et al. 2004. Cognitive-behavioral therapy for anger in children and adolescents: a meta-analysis. *Aggress Violent Behav*, 9, 247–69.

Sukhodolsky, D. G., et al. 2009. Randomized trial of anger control training for adolescents with Tourette's syndrome and disruptive behavior. *J Am Acad Child Adolesc Psychiatry*, 48, 413–21.

Surguladze, S. A., et al. 2003. A preferential increase in the extrastriate response to signals of danger. *NeuroImage*, 19, 1317–28.

Surman, C. B., et al. 2011. Deficient emotional self-regulation and adult attention deficit hyperactivity disorder: a family risk analysis. *Am J Psychiatry*, 168, 617–23.

Talarovicova, A., et al. 2007. Some assessments of the amygdala role in suprahypothalamic neuroendocrine regulation: a minireview. *Endocr Regul*, 41, 155–62.

Tateno, A., et al. 2003. Clinical correlates of aggressive behavior after traumatic brain injury. *J Neuropsychiat Clin Neurosci*, 15, 155–60.

Taylor, E., et al. 1984. Hyperactive behavior in English schoolchildren: a questionnaire survey. *J Abnorm Child Psychol*, 12, 143–55.

Taylor, E., et al. 1991. *The epidemiology of childhood hyperactivity*. Oxford: Oxford University Press.

Taylor, E., et al. 2008. Disorders of attention and activity. In: Rutter, M., Bishop, D. V. M., Pine, D. S., Scott, S., Stevenson, J., Taylor, E., & and Thapar, A. (eds), *Rutter's child and adolescent psychiatry*, 5th edn, pp. 521–42. Oxford: Blackwell Publishing.

Tohen, M., et al. 2007. Olanzapine versus placebo in the treatment of adolescents with bipolar mania. *Am J Psychiatry*, 164, 1547–56.

Tramontina, S., et al. 2009. Aripiprazole in children and adolescents with bipolar disorder comorbid with attention-deficit/hyperactivity disorder: a pilot randomized clinical trial. *J Clin Psychiatry*, 70, 756–64.

Troost, P. W., et al. 2005. Long-term effects of risperidone in children with autism spectrum disorders: a placebo discontinuation study. *J Am Acad Child Adolesc Psychiatry*, 44, 1137–44.

Wagner, K. D., et al. 2002. An open-label trial of divalproex in children and adolescents with bipolar disorder. *J Am Acad Child Adolesc Psychiatry*, 41, 1224–30.

Wakschlag, L. S., et al. 2007. A developmental framework for distinguishing disruptive behavior from normative misbehavior in preschool children. *J Child Psychol Psychiatry*, 48, 976–87.

Wakschlag, L. S., et al. 2010. Research review: 'Ain't misbehavin'': towards a developmentally-specified nosology for preschool disruptive behavior. *J Child Psychol Psychiatry*, 51, 3–22.

Wakschlag, L. S., et al. 2012. Defining the developmental parameters of temper loss in early childhood: implications for developmental psychopathology. *J Child Psychol Psychiatry*, 53, 1099–108.

Wasman, M., et al. 1962. Directed attack elicited from hypothalamus. *Arch Neurol*, 6, 220–7.

Weissman, M. M., et al. 1971. Clinical evaluation of hostility in depression. *Am J Psychiatry*, 128, 261–6.

Wierzbicka, A. 1999. Emotion universals. *Language Design*, 2, 23–69.

Wilkowski, B. M., et al. 2008. The cognitive basis of trait anger and reactive aggression: an integrative analysis. *Pers Soc Psychol Rev*, 12, 3–21.

Wittchen, H. U., et al. 1998. Prevalence of mental disorders and psychosocial impairments in adolescents and young adults. *Psychol Med*, 28, 109–26.

Woolfenden, S. R., et al. 2001. Family and parenting interventions in children and adolescents with conduct disorder and delinquency aged 10–17. *Cochrane Database Syst Rev*, (2):CD003015.

Wozniak, J., et al. 1995. Mania-like symptoms suggestive of childhood-onset bipolar disorder in clinically referred children. *J Am Acad Child Adolesc Psychiatry*, 34, 867–76.

Yatham, L. N., et al. 2005. Canadian Network for Mood and Anxiety Treatments (CANMAT) guidelines for the management of patients with bipolar disorder: consensus and controversies. *Bipolar Disord*, 3, 5–69.

Yudofsky, S. C., et al. 1986. The Overt Aggression Scale for the objective rating of verbal and physical aggression. *Am J Psychiatry*, 143, 35–9.

Zahn-Waxler, C., et al. 1996. Japanese and United States preschool children's responses to conflict and distress. *Child Dev*, 67, 2462–77.

Zahreddine, N. Stringaris, A. 2014. *Treatment of Bipolar Disorder in children and adolescents*. In Maudsley Prescribing Guidelines 12th Edition, Editors David Taylor and Shittij Kapur. John Wiley & Sons.

Zuddas, A., et al. 2000. Long-term risperidone for pervasive developmental disorder: efficacy, tolerability, and discontinuation. *J Child Adolesc Psychopharmacol*, 10, 79–90.

Index